Cross-Cultural Medicine

Cross-Cultural Medicine

EDITED BY

JudyAnn Bigby, MD

Associate Professor of Medicine
Harvard Medical School
Brigham and Women's Hospital
Boston, Massachusetts

American College of Physicians / Philadelphia

Manager, Book Publishing: David Myers
Acquisitions Editor: Mary K. Ruff
Developmental Editor: Victoria Hoenigke
Production Supervisor: Allan S. Kleinberg
Editorial Assistant: Alicia Dillihay
Designer: Kate Nichols
Indexer: Nelle Garrecht

Printed in the United States of America
Composition by UB Communications
Printing/binding by Versa Press

American College of Physicians (ACP) became an imprint of the American College of Physicians–American Society of Internal Medicine in July 1998.

Library of Congress Cataloging-in-Publication Data

Cross-cultural medicine / [edited by] JudyAnn Bigby.
    p. ; cm.
    Includes bibliographical references and index.
    ISBN 1-930513-02-X
    1. Transcultural medical care. 2. Minorities—Medical care. 3. Social medicine. 4. Ethnic groups—Health and hygiene. I. Bigby, JudyAnn. II. American College of Physicians—American Society of Internal Medicine.
    [DNLM: 1. Delivery of Health Care—methods—United States. 2. Ethnic Groups—United States. 3. Cross–Cultural Comparison—United States. 4. Cultural Diversity—United States. 5. Health Behavior—ethnology—United States. 6. Minority Groups—United States. WA 300 C9515 2002]
    RA418.5.T73.C765 2002
    613'.089—dc21

                              2002074652

03 04 05 06 07 / 9 8 7 6 5 4 3 2 1

2/11/04

To my patients
who have taught me so much

Contributors

Linda Barnes, PhD, MTS, MA
Assistant Professor
Boston University School of
    Medicine
Boston, Massachusetts

JudyAnn Bigby, MD, MPH
Associate Professor of Medicine
Harvard Medical School
Brigham and Women's Hospital
Boston, Massachusetts

Jean Lau Chin, EdD
CEO Services – Clinical-Educational-
    Organizational Services
Newton, Massachusetts

**Christine Makosky Daley, MA,
    SM**
Candidate and Lecturer
Department of Anthropology
University of Connecticut
Storrs, Connecticut

Sean M. Daley, MA
Candidate and Lecturer
Department of Anthropology
University of Connecticut
Storrs, Connecticut

Maya M. Hammoud, MD
Director of Middle Eastern Women's
    Health Program
University of Michigan Medical Center
Women's Hospital
Ann Arbor, Michigan

Susana Morales, MD
Associate Professor of Clinical Medicine
Associate Chair for Educational Affairs
Weill Medical College
Cornell University
New York, New York

Barbara Ogur, MD
Assistant Professor of Medicine
Department of Medicine
Harvard Medical School and
    Cambridge Health Alliance
Cambridge, Massachusetts

M. Kay Siblani, RN
President, CEO, and Consultant
Oasis Communications, Inc.
Dearborn Heights, Michigan

Melissa Welch, MD, MPH
Associate Clinical Professor
University of California, San Francisco
San Francisco, California

Contents

I

Beyond Culture: Strategies for Caring for Patients from Diverse Racial, Ethnic, and Cultural Groups

JUDYANN BIGBY, MD

ross-Cultural Medicine presents internists with a framework for practicing culturally competent care. It provides important background information on various racial, ethnic, and cultural groups common in the United States, provides an overview of typical health problems facing those groups, and describes common approaches to enhancing care. The reader should consider the various chapters devoted to each group not as specific treatments for care but rather as a foundation for exploring an individual's health beliefs and concerns in the context of his or her sociocultural experiences.

It is important for physicians to have a common language when exploring issues of culture, race, and ethnicity in the medical setting. Throughout this book the terms *race* and *ethnicity* are used in a consistent fashion (see below). Though the term *minority* has a negative connotation to many individuals, used here it refers to the numeric size of one group relative to another larger racial or ethnic group, usually whites. In some areas of the country minority group populations collectively are becoming the majority population.

Terms and Concepts

Race refers to historical anthropological categories of people. The United States government uses the following racial categories: American Indian/Alaska Native, Asian American, African American or black, Native Hawaiian/Pacific Islander, white. Historically most racial classifications acknowledged at least three major categories: Caucasian, Negro, and Mongoloid; these terms are now outdated. As many as 16 racial categories have been proposed (1). Interestingly, 70% of Hispanics would prefer to have *Hispanic* considered a racial category (2).

One definition from the public health literature recognizes race as a social construct that originates from societal desire to separate people based on their looks and culture, *race* being considered a vague, unscientific term referring to a group of genetically related individuals who share certain physical characteristics.

Despite an ostensible genetic similarity within a race, there is not necessarily a biological distinctiveness between people of different races.

Ethnicity describes certain subgroups that share ancestry, history, or culture. Factors that bind members of an ethnic group are diverse and include, but are not limited to, geographic origin (e.g., Middle Eastern, West Indian, Southerners), language or dialect, culture (music, literature, culinary habits), religion, and gender roles. The United States government classifies Hispanics as an ethnic group that may be of any race. Some members of this group prefer the term *Latino*.

Culture may be defined as a shared system of values, beliefs, and learned patterns of behavior. Professional status may affect culture (e.g., "medical culture"). For the purposes of the discussion in this chapter, culture includes racial and ethnic characteristics.

Acknowledging that race is a social rather than biological construct whose meaning can and has changed over time is not to dismiss the importance of race or racial identity. Ethnicity, nationality, or class does not subsume racial category. As discussed by Williams (2), racial categories reflect the importance of race in United States history and the inequalities arising out of the treatment of people according to their race. People who appear to be of African descent are often treated in a certain way regardless of their ethnicity, nationality, or social class. Race categorization is reflected in American society in a way that ethnicity, culture, and class are not: "Race . . . is a determinant of access to society's rewards and resources" (2). Though concepts of race and ethnicity may overlap, they are not interchangeable categories.

Why is Cultural Competence Important?

Changing Demographics

Between 1990 and 2000, the United States population significantly changed. The percentage of non-Hispanic whites in the population decreased from

80% to 75%. The black population increased from 12.1% to 12.9%, the Hispanic population from 9% to 12.5%, and the Asian/Pacific Islander population from 2.8% to nearly 3.6%, while the American Indian/Alaska Native population remained steady at just under 1% (3). Though the total population became more diverse during the 1990s, the physician population did not keep pace. Underrepresented minority groups (African American, mainland Puerto Rican, Mexican American, American Indian/Alaska Native) represent approximately 11% of first-year medical students but more than 25% of the United States population (4). Other minority groups (e.g., Central and South American) are also underrepresented in medical schools. Some ethnic and racial minority groups (e.g., Asian Indian, Chinese American, other Asian American) are increasingly represented among medical school classes and play an important role in delivering care to underserved populations (5). Most physicians practicing today are white, however, and there is the possibility of racial and ethnic discordance between the physician and patient in most regions of the country. This discordance is most pronounced in the southern United States where a high percentage of African Americans live, in the Southwest with a large population of Latino residents, and in the West with a large population of Asian and Latino residents. Other parts of the country are home to certain immigrant groups, such as the Middle Eastern and Arab population around Detroit, the Southeast Asian population in parts of Minnesota, and the Dominican and Central American population in parts of the Northeast. These groups are also unlikely to be able to see physicians representative of their race, ethnicity, or culture.

Between 1990 and 2000 the American population grew by 32.7 million people, the largest census-to-census increase in American history. According to the 2000 census, nearly 10% of the population was foreign born. The Census Bureau estimates that by the year 2050 the white non-Hispanic population will decrease to 52.8%; the black non-Hispanic population will remain stable at about 13%; the Native Alaskan/American Indian population will remain stable at just under 1%; the Asian population will increase to nearly 8.2%; and the Hispanic population will increase to 24.5% (Fig. 1-1). These data are compelling reasons in themselves for all physicians to become more versed in the social circumstances, cultural beliefs, and unique health concerns of minority group and immigrant populations, but other reasons exist as well.

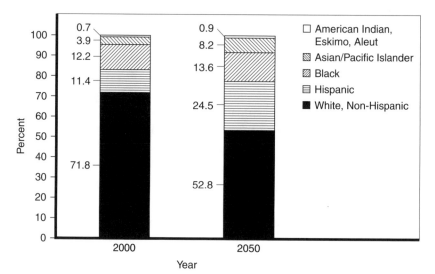

Source: Bureau of the Census, Decennial Census and Population Projections.

Figure 1-1   Percent of population by race and Hispanic origin, 2000 and 2050 (projected).

Disparities in Health Status

Over the last two decades researchers have documented in more than 600 citations disparities in access to care and health status for individuals from racial and ethnic minority groups in the United States. In 1985 Secretary of Health and Human Services Margaret Heckler first documented the extent of these disparities in Report of the Secretary's Task Force on Black and Minority Health (6). Recently former Surgeon General David Satcher drew attention to ongoing, and in some cases increasing, racial and ethnic disparities in health status, particularly infant mortality, heart disease, HIV/AIDS, diabetes, cancer, and immunizations. A major goal of Healthy People 2010 is to eliminate health disparities (7). Unfortunately, disparities are most pronounced for the racial and ethnic minority groups that are among the fastest growing populations. Therefore the future health of America will be influenced substantially by the health of those from racial and ethnic minority groups.

An important study by the Henry J. Kaiser Family Foundation in 1999 suggested that the American public may not be specifically aware of racial and ethnic disparities in health status indicators such as infant mortality and life expectancy (8). However, the study demonstrated that individuals from racial and ethnic minority groups, specifically blacks and Latinos, perceive that they receive a lower quality of health care than whites in the United States. A significant proportion also reported that they had been discriminated against because of their financial or health insurance status, because of their race or ethnicity, and because of their uncertain or poor use of the English language. Though a significant percentage of whites also reported bias or disrespect in the health care system due to their financial or health insurance status, they were significantly less likely to report this experience than black or Latino respondents.

According to a report from the Commonwealth Fund (9), blacks, Hispanics, and Asian Americans are more likely to report difficulty accessing health care, paying for medications and other out-of-pocket expenses, and identifying a regular physician. A growing body of evidence has documented disparities in access to procedures such as cardiac catheterization, joint replacement, screening procedures such as mammography, immunizations, and kidney transplants. In addition, the prevalence of chronic disease is significantly higher among some racial or ethnic groups. For example, diabetes is two to four times more prevalent in black, Hispanics, and Native American women than it is among white women; Hepatitis B and tuberculosis are more prevalent among Asian Americans; and infant mortality rates are still 2.5 to 3 times higher for black infants than for white infants. Not all groups in the United States have enjoyed the same degree of advancement in life expectancy and decreases in deaths from cardiac disease and cancer (10). While these disparities may not be caused by inadequate or below-standard physician care, physicians *can* play a role in decreasing disparities by being aware of them, examining their own behavior, and helping to advocate for health care systems that address and eliminate rather than promote disparities. Eliminating disparities should be a key outcome of delivering culturally competent care.

What Accounts for Racial and Ethnic Health Disparities?

Many factors contribute to racial and ethnic health disparities. These include genetic or biologic differences, social factors such as education and income, personal beliefs and attitudes that determine specific health behaviors and behaviors that influence risk, interpersonal relations with providers and individual provider behavior, and health care policies and procedures.

These factors do not influence health status independently but interact in a complicated fashion (Fig. 1-2).

There is increasing evidence that the gene pool is not significantly different across racial and ethnic groups. Race is not a biologically or anthropologically sound concept. It appears that the genetic makeup of all individuals is more homogenous than heterogeneous. Some of the observed differences based on race and ethnicity may be due to extrinsic factors. For example, the increased prevalence of the *BRCA-1* gene among Jewish Ashkenazi women compared with the general population may be related to the relative geographic and cultural isolation of this group. Other apparent biological differences (e.g., differences in drug receptors and metabolism of different substances) reflect differences in the distribution of polymorphic gene traits (11). Biologic differences alone cannot account for the observed disparities.

Individual characteristics such as income, education, and occupation as well as factors such as immigration status, housing, geographic location, and social/political standing define one's socioeconomic status. Community characteristics such as environment (natural and man-made), quality of schools, and safety also influence health status. Lower socioeconomic status *is* associated with poorer health; however, although the influence of

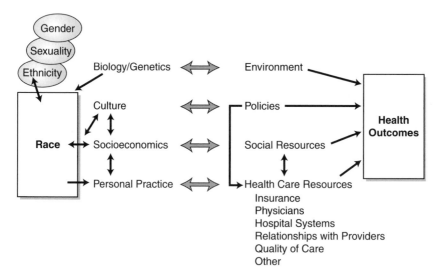

Figure 1-2 Factors contributing to racial and ethnic health disparities. These factors interact with each other on multiple levels.

socioeconomic status cannot be denied, it in itself is inadequate to explain all racial and ethnic disparities. For example, the disparity in infant mortality between black and white infants is actually higher between black and white women with at least a high school education than between black and white women with less education.

Individual behavior and personal beliefs also are important contributors to health status. Some policy makers estimate that 50% of health outcomes are determined by an individual's behavior as it relates to smoking, diet, exercise, sexual activity, exposure to guns, and use of drugs and alcohol (12). This concept is most appropriate for understanding the health of various populations as opposed to individuals. Individuals acquire behaviors, including health behaviors, in the context of their sociocultural and sociopolitical circumstances. Patients do not act independently of physicians and other providers. Their health care decisions are influenced by past experiences in the health care system, including relations with physicians, and other factors that cannot be completely separated from personal behavior.

Several studies suggest that physician behavior may contribute to disparities in health due to differential treatment, lack of recognition of different presenting signs and symptoms, and less time spent with patients (13,14). Studies demonstrate that physician behavior influences, in particular, mammography screening for black and Latino women, referral for invasive cardiac procedures, and treatment with analgesics.

Institutional policies and procedures may also affect the health outcomes of minority patients. Location, hours of operation, availability of interpreters, and availability of key written materials in languages other than English can influence access to health care and the quality of diagnosis and treatment.

What is Cultural Competence?

Cultural competence is a means, not an end. Cultural competence is the ability of health care providers and institutions to deliver effective services to racially, ethnically, and culturally diverse patient populations. Some physicians are culturally competent (at most times); others are not (or rarely). There are several key components of cultural competence: personal self-awareness, cultural knowledge, ability to perform a cultural assessment, understanding and recognition of the dynamics of difference, effective communication, and cultural desire (internal motivation).

Personal Self-Awareness

Personal self-awareness is an essential element of cultural competence. The concept of physicians learning about the health beliefs and exotic health behaviors of "others" to achieve cultural competence is limiting and reinforces stereotypes, blames others for their conditions, and leaves unattended issues of intentional or unintentional discrimination or bias. Acknowledging one's personal identity or, more accurately, identities, is an important first step in developing cultural competence. Understanding how one's own race, ethnicity, culture, socioeconomic status, sexual orientation, and other characteristics influences one's practice as a physician can help to expose sources of one's own beliefs and biases. To understand how they relate to other individuals, physicians must first understand themselves.

Personal self-reflection and self-critique are required to explore how different life experiences influence interactions with patients. The experience of an individual physician is determined by his or her family, community, and personal experience in the health care system. Individuals who have had little exposure to the groups of patients for whom they eventually provide health care may have learned or been influenced to hold specific beliefs about those groups that are based on stereotypes. These stereotypes may have been learned from, or reinforced by, movies, music, television, newspapers, or books, or an isolated incident with an individual from that particular group.

Self-reflection is an important process for developing personal self-awareness. Individual physicians may engage in a number of personal exercises to facilitate self-reflection. The questions in Box 1-1 represent a sample of the types of issues physicians can explore in this process (15). By reviewing the questions and reflecting on their responses, physicians can gain a better understanding of why they may have more success with some patients than with others in building relationships, recommending appropriate therapies, and achieving successful outcomes.

Physicians may choose to explore these questions with colleagues with whom they feel comfortable. Participation in discussion groups that use literature or movies to identify key concepts may also be an effective means of identifying sources of bias and in understanding one's own cultural beliefs.

Box 1-1 Questions for Assessing Cultural Self-Awareness

1. How do you define your own racial or ethnic identity?
2. What did you learn to value while you were growing up?
3. What are some of the features of your own racial or ethnic group that you view positively?
4. What are some of the features of your own racial or ethnic group that you view negatively?
5. While you were growing up were the schools and neighborhoods homogenous or racially and/or ethnically mixed? At what point in your life did you have the opportunity to interact with people who were different from you?
6. Are there other racial or ethnic groups with which you feel comfortable?
7. Are there other racial or ethnic groups with which you feel uncomfortable?
8. What is the racial/ethnic or socio-cultural characteristic of the patients with whom you feel most competent in establishing rapport and establishing a treatment plan?
9. What is the racial/ethnic or socio-cultural characteristic of patients with whom you have the most difficulty establishing rapport and establishing a treatment plan?
10. How do factors related to your racial or ethnic identity and/or from your life experience affect how you interact with patients from backgrounds that are different from your own?

Adapted from Goldman R, Monroe AD, Dube C. Ann Behav Sci Med Educ. 1996;3:37-46.

Writing a journal about one's cultural beliefs and outlooks may be a useful self-analytical tool.

Another key concept physicians should explore in their process of self-reflection is the role of power in the doctor/patient relationship. Historically physicians have had hierarchical relationships with patients. When there is discordance due to characteristics such as gender, socioeconomic status, race, ethnicity, and sexual orientation between the doctor and patient, the differential in power between the doctor and patient can be magnified and lead to inappropriate use of power to establish treatment priorities and articulate desirable outcomes. Pinderhughes (16) suggests that providers explore how the power differential plays out by reflecting on circumstances when they have felt different because of personal characteristics and when they have felt powerless because of this difference. Alternatively physicians can reflect on situations when they acknowledge their power and how they use it.

Cultural Knowledge

Cultural knowledge includes not only knowledge of key aspects of a patient's cultural beliefs but also an awareness of historical perspective (the history that may shape certain beliefs and attitudes) (see Chapter 7), cultural context (the cultural norms that shape health behaviors [e.g., the role of the family in decision making]), and epidemiologic and biological expressions of disease and response to treatment. Physicians should not only be aware of different cultural beliefs or concepts of health and illness but also become skilled in exploring how or whether these beliefs are important or relevant to a specific individual. Common concepts of disease etiology are explored further in this book.

Some cultural beliefs regarding illness causation include theories regarding conditions of the blood ("high blood" versus "low blood," "bad blood," "thin blood" versus "thick blood"), imbalances in nature and the body (hot/cold theories), and stress or other emotional states (17). Becoming familiar with such beliefs may be useful but does not replace the need to investigate the importance of the specific health beliefs of the individual patient. In addition, physicians should recognize that in different populations certain signs and symptoms are assigned significance that influence perception of disease. Pain, weight loss, or fever may be viewed by the patient as symptoms that warrant immediate and thorough investigation or treatment. Understanding the significance of these symptoms in certain cultures has implications for how to approach a problem with certain patients (e.g., fever and respiratory symptoms may be particularly anxiety provoking in Puerto Ricans and feeling weak particularly anxiety provoking in Haitians).

Understanding the historical or sociocultural context of an individual or the group with which an individual identifies is important. The Tuskegee syphilis experiment is often cited as an example of how black Americans came to distrust the American health care system (18). For 40 years the Public Health Service conducted a study of untreated syphilis on black men in Alabama. These men were told that they had "bad blood," which has several connotations among people in the rural South, including infection or contamination. Even after penicillin was accepted as an effective and safe treatment for syphilis, the men were not treated. The female partners of the men were not informed of the infection and also went untreated. The study was no secret; the results were widely published in medical journals. Only after an employee of the Public Health Service went to the press to express his concerns about the unethical nature of the experiment and its poor scientific design did the study end. An apology from the federal government was not forthcoming to the victims and their families until more than 20 years later.

Less frequently discussed racial injustices, such as the forced sterilization of some black and poor women, also can have an impact on health-seeking behaviors. At a health forum for community women an African American physician discussed disparities in breast cancer deaths among black women. A member of the audience volunteered that black women do not like to get mammograms "because we don't like to be touched. We had our bodies invaded when we didn't want them invaded so it's hard to go for a test when you know some stranger is going to touch your breasts."

Case 1-1 illustrates what happens when historical perspectives, ethnic concepts of disease, and individual factors that influence health beliefs intersect. Obviously in this case the word "contaminated" had different meanings for the physician and the patient. The concept of a contaminated blood culture is foreign to most patients. The implications of having contaminated blood were significant for this patient. The lack of a clear explanation of the meaning of contaminated blood culture from the physician caused much distress for the patient and eroded her confidence in the health care system.

The sociocultural context of individual health care experiences is influenced by group values and norms. Table 1-1 provides a summary of some common cultural norms for different racial and ethnic groups and for the medical construct (biomedical systems); it is adapted from the work of Dr Edwin Nichols (19). Issues such as how time is viewed, which relationships are valued, and how knowledge is obtained can have a profound impact on the doctor/patient relationship. Understanding how individuals value these particular entities helps physicians address such issues as appointments, taking medications, and preventive behaviors. Case 1-2 illustrates what can happen when physicians and patients are operating under different value systems and assumptions.

CASE 1-1   A 70-YEAR-OLD BLACK WOMAN DIAGNOSED WITH "BAD BLOOD"

Mrs Jackson is a 70-year-old black woman who has lived in the Northeast for 36 years after moving from Alabama. She presented to the emergency department with shortness of breath and chest discomfort. She was found to have congestive heart failure and uncontrolled hypertension. During her emergency room assessment, blood cultures were drawn for unclear reasons. One blood culture grew Staphylococcus epidermidis. The physician in charge, who was not her regular physician, relayed this result to Mrs Jackson. He told her the blood culture was contaminated and she should not be concerned.

Two weeks later Mrs Jackson returned to the outpatient department to see her long-standing primary care physician. She was distraught over her hospitalization. After much discussion her physician ascertained that Mrs Jackson was upset because she had been told that her blood was contaminated. She believed that this was the same as having "bad blood," a sexually transmitted disease.

Mrs Jackson, a very religious widow, was offended that the physician in the hospital had thought she had "bad blood." She demanded to see her medical record to make sure that any reference to her blood being contaminated was deleted from the chart. She was not satisfied with the medical definition of contaminated blood culture offered by her primary care physician. She became concerned that she had been injected with bacteria, especially because no one could give a clear reason why she had had a blood culture taken. Mrs Jackson transferred her care to another institution.

In spite of the growing evidence that there is less variation in the human genome across racial groups than within racial groups, important differences exist in epidemiologic patterns of disease, physiologic manifestations, and response to treatment across racial groups. Genetic factors or external factors such as diet or the environment may account for these differences.

Table 1-1 Different Cultural Concepts of Relationships, Time, and Knowledge Acquisition

	Euro-American	African American/Latino	Asian American	Biomedical Systems
Values	• Man-to-object • Personal control over environment • Individualism • Privacy • Master of own fate	• Man-to-man • High context communication • Birthright, inheritance • Interpersonal relatedness • Community	• Man-to-group • Group welfare • Cohesiveness of group • Interdependence • Hierarchy, rank	• Man-to-object • Personal control over disease • Disease as an object to be cured • Personal responsibility
Time	• Future oriented	• Relaxed with time • Past oriented • Oriented to situation	• Harmony with nature • Past and future connected • Fatalism • Karmic ties • Tradition	• Linear orientation
How knowledge is acquired; how to come to know	• Counting and measuring • Understanding relation of parts to whole • Action • Goal setting • Work orientation	• Seeing the whole • Symbolic imagery and rhythms • Spiritualism • Mathematics as it relates biorhythm	• Transcendental • Parts and whole considered together • Small sample studied thoroughly and connected to universe	• Counting and measuring • Quantifying (e.g., size of lesions, amount of drugs, levels of drugs, rates of cure)

Adapted from a private communication from Edwin Nichols.

Racial differences in drug metabolism or drug effects have been described for beta-blockers, warfarin, angiotension-converting enzyme inhibitors, anti-depressants, alcohol, and nicotine, to name a few.

Cultural Assessment

The ability to incorporate a *cultural assessment* into the various aspects of clinical encounters with patients is an important feature of cultural competence.

CASE 1-2   A 28-YEAR-OLD DOMINICAN WOMAN WHO
MISSES APPOINTMENTS

Ms Cortazar is a 28-year-old Dominican woman who has lived in the United States for 14 years. She has 2 children, ages 7 and 9. She had an abnormal Pap smear, showing ASCUS, 6 months ago. She is scheduled for a repeat Pap smear. Her appointment is at 2:30 and she arrives 90 min early. She waits until 2 o'clock and is not seen. She observes that two women who arrived after her are taken in before her. At 2:10 she abruptly leaves the clinic. Her provider calls her at home and explains how important it is to have her repeat Pap smear. She agrees to schedule another appointment.

Two weeks later she arrives for her 3 o'clock appointment at 3:55. She waits until 4:30 until her provider calls her in. The provider in turn is clearly annoyed that she was late for her appointment and does the Pap smear in an abrupt fashion. When Ms Cortazar asks when the results will be available, the provider says he will send her the results whenever he gets them. She overhears him telling the nurse that he will not see her again if she arrives so late for her appointment. As she leaves, Ms Cortazar announces to the secretary that she is not coming back to the clinic because of the way she has been treated.

DISCUSSION

Ms Cortazar is trying to juggle her roles as mother and part-time worker with her responsibility for her own health. She works in the morning as a manager in a local pharmacy. She has no after-school care for her children and must be at home when they arrive from school. This makes it difficult for her to keep a medical appointment in the afternoon. If she leaves work in the morning she will lose pay, because she is paid by the hour. She believed that if she arrived early for her appointment she would be seen before her scheduled time and would then be able to get home before her children arrived from school. She arrived late for her second appointment because she waited for her children to arrive home from school and had to make sure that her friend was available to look after them.

The physician does not understand why someone would arrive so early for an appointment and then leave without being seen. The patient was not asked nor did she volunteer an explanation. After Ms Cortazar arrived late for the second appointment, the physician was understandably irritated but, again, did not question the patient as to the reason.

This case is a classic example of how two people may have different concepts of time. For the physician, the appointment time was firm. For the patient, the appointment time was flexible. She first assumed the doctor would see her before the scheduled time if she arrived early, then assumed that if she were an hour late the physician would not mind. These misunderstandings were compounded by lack of communication.

How could this unfortunate situation have been avoided? The physician could have begun by telling Ms Cortazar how important it was to him that patients arrive on time. He could have considerately asked her if she had some special circumstances that made it difficult for her to keep appointments. For instance, "You arrived very early for your last appointment, then left before being seen, and today you were late. Is there a problem with your appointment times? With transportation? Personal reasons?" This opens the door for a discussion of the patient's personal circumstances and values. This can lead to more trust between the two so that in the future the patient may be willing to bring her problems directly to the provider or secretary.

Cultural assessments extend beyond an ascertainment of a patient's specific health beliefs and can provide physicians with important information about the patient's sociocultural context. Physicians cannot assume they "know" a patient based only on observations of race or knowledge of the patient's language or country or geographic area of origin. For example, describing a patient as black does not reveal anything about the person's self-identity. Black Americans born in the United States may all be considered "African American" but may have different health beliefs and experiences depending on whether they are from a rural or urban background. Blacks who have immigrated to the United States may have come from the many different islands in the Caribbean or from Africa. These individuals will have different cultures and health care beliefs and experiences. Black women who have immigrated to the United States have better pregnancy outcomes than American-born black women, which suggests that the experience of being a black American is an important condition for poor birth outcomes.

Describing an individual as Spanish speaking is even less revealing. Individuals who classify themselves as Latino may also identify themselves as Puerto Rican and come from the Island or from the mainland United States. Latinos also come from a variety of diverse areas including the Caribbean, Central America, and South America. As with blacks, Latino within-group diversity is significant.

Understanding the cultural context of individuals requires physicians to know something about a patient's level of formal education, income, religion, and occupation. The physician may also want to know how connected the patient is to his or her community. Performing a cultural assessment often requires that physicians allow patients to use a narrative style to relay information as opposed to having patients answer specific questions. For example:

- "Tell me about yourself and your family."
- "How have you come to be in this part of the United States?"
- "Tell me about your past experiences in the health care system. Does anything stand out?"

Physicians who have ongoing relationships with patients will have the opportunity to perform this assessment over many visits and therefore should not feel pressured to obtain all the background material immediately. In fact, physicians may find that they are better able to obtain this information over weeks and months as patients develop trust and a certain comfort level with their physicians.

Physicians must be able to assess an individual patient's values and beliefs and to incorporate this information into clinical assessments and decision-making. Physicians may use a general framework for issues that are important to specific groups to guide their interviews with patients, but they must avoid making assumptions about individual behaviors and risks, personal preferences, and social context and confirm their impressions through direct inquiries. Box 1-2 provides strategies and key content areas for clinical cultural assessments. Physicians can inquire about this information briefly while taking the social history and in more detail as they establish rapport with patients.

The Dynamics of Difference

Accepting that difference exists between physicians and patients is an important step in developing cultural competence. Physicians who accept that different attitudes, expectations, and health beliefs may exist between themselves and their patients will have an easier time exploring the role difference plays in the patient/doctor interaction. It is also important to understand that the physician and patient will experience the same situation from different perspectives based on their individual assumptions about each other and their previous experiences in society at large and in the heath care system.

Suggesting that difference does not matter is an expression of cultural blindness. In this circumstance, physicians assert that they treat all people alike regardless of race or culture. Though this view may be well intentioned, it disregards reality and in actuality requires patients who are racially and ethnically different from the more prevalent culture to assimilate towards that culture. Their personal beliefs and values are not acknowledged and therefore not valued or considered in the context of eliciting their expectations of the health care system, understanding their complaints or symptoms, and devising a diagnostic or treatment strategy.

Understanding and accepting differences between the doctor and the patient is important for achieving certain measures of quality of care. For example, patient satisfaction may be influenced by this parameter. If patients have different expectations for how providers demonstrate respect (e.g., whether a physician addresses an individual by first name or by surname), physicians can inadvertently express disrespect for one group of patients.

Effective Communication

Communication skills are an essential component of cultural competence. Even when a patient speaks the same language as the physician,

Box 1-2   Strategies and Key Content Areas for Clinical Cultural Assessments

Strategies*

- Consider all patients as individuals first.
- Do not assume that ethnic identity indicates specific cultural values or behavior.
- Consider all generalizations about cultural norms for specific groups as hypotheses, then test them.
- Most people from racial and ethnic minority groups are, by necessity, bicultural in American society; the degree of acclimatization varies.
- Some aspects of a patient's cultural history, values, and beliefs are relevant to clinical situations and some are not. Do not prejudge which are relevant; let the patient tell you
- Identify strategies taken from the patient's cultural orientation that you both can use to enhance the therapeutic alliance. Acknowledge those that seem counter-productive.
- Familiarize yourself with interactional norms:
  - ➤ Age (how younger clinicians should show respect for elders; how older clinicians should encourage young patients to ask questions or express opinion)
  - ➤ Across gender
  - ➤ Across class

Content†

Over time or as appropriate for the situation investigate the five factors that seem to independently contribute to health behavior:
- Exposure to biomedical and popular standards of care as determined by
  - ➤ Level of formal education
  - ➤ Generational status
  - ➤ Level of encapsulation within ethnic and family social network
  - ➤ Experience of medical treatment
  - ➤ Previous experience with particular diseases
  - ➤ Age at immigration (if applicable)
  - ➤ Degree of migration back and forth to country of origin (if applicable)
- Income
- Occupation
- Area of origin in native country (if applicable)
- Religion

* Adapted from DiversityRx Web site at www.diversityRx.org.
† For more detailed discussion see, for example, Harwood A. Guidelines for culturally appropriate health care. In: Harwood A, ed. Ethnicity and Medical Care. Cambridge, MA: Harvard University Press; 1981:483-507.

communication between a doctor and a patient may be ineffective if personal characteristics such as race, educational status, and cultural background are not acknowledged and taken into account. Excellent communication requires effective speaking, listening, and observation.

Several educators have developed models that describe the various components of effective cross-cultural/racial/ethnic communication. Berlin and Fowkes (21) use the acronym LEARN to describe several key skills (Box 1-3). In the LEARN model listening is the first step to effective cross-cultural/racial/ethnic communication. Listening to the patient's perspective requires that physicians have an effective strategy for eliciting the patient's explanatory model of illness. Kleinman and colleagues (22) have suggested several questions based on an anthropologic approach. When asked in a respectful, caring manner these questions can facilitate an understanding of the patient's expectations and provide important facts that may not come up in a traditional medical interview. Beginning with an explanation about why a physician might ask these questions helps to establish a respectful atmosphere and demonstrates genuine interest in the response. For instance:

> I know that patients and doctors sometimes have different ideas about diseases and what causes them, so I think it's important for the doctor to get a clear idea about what the patient thinks. That's why I'd like to know more about your ideas about the disease or problem that we have been discussing.

Physicians should be able to identify discrepancies between their concepts of disease and the patient's. As described in the LEARN model, the physician must be able to effectively explain the basis for his or her assessment of the patient's concerns and explain how his or her explanation differs from the patient's. This requires that the physician acknowledge the patient's explanatory model and point out the similarities and differences between his or her explanation. In some instances the patient's model can be incorporated into the physician's. The physician should offer his recommendations for the next steps in a manner the patient can understand. If the patient is hesitant, explore the source of hesitation and begin to negotiate a mutually agreed upon plan.

The Diversity Curriculum Task Force of the Boston University Residency Program in Internal Medicine has developed a model for care, using

Box 1-3   Different Approaches to Effective Cross-Cultural Racial/Ethnic Communication

LEARN*

Listen to the patient's perspective.

Explain and share one's own perspective.

Acknowledge differences and similarities between two perspectives.

Recommend treatment.

Negotiate mutually agreed upon plan.

Eliciting the Patient's Explanatory Model of Illness†

• What do you call your illness?

• When did your illness begin?

• Why do you think your illness started?

• How severe is your illness?

• What do you fear most about your illness?

• What are the major problems your illness has caused?

• Do you have any ideas about what treatment you should receive?

• Can you think of any specialists who may be helpful?

RESPECT‡

Respect—A demonstrable attitude involving both verbal and nonverbal communications

Explanatory model—What is the patient's point of view about his or her illness? How does it relate to the physician's point of view? All points of view must be elicited and reconciled.

Sociocultural context—How class, race, ethnicity, gender, education, sexual orientation, immigrant status, and family and gender roles, for example, affect care

Power—Acknowledging the power differential between patients and physicians

Empathy—Putting into words the significance of the patient's concerns so that he or she feels understood by the physician

Concerns and fears—Eliciting the patient's emotions and concerns

Therapeutic alliance/Trust—A measurable outcome that enhances adherence to, and engagement in, health care

---

* LEARN model developed by Berlin EA, Fowkes WC. A teaching framework for cross-cultural health care. West J Med. 1983;139:935.

† Adapted from Kleinman A, Eisenberg L, Good B. Culture, illness, and care: clinical lessons from anthropologic and cross-cultural research. Ann Intern Med. 1978;88:251-8.

‡ RESPECT model developed by the Boston University Residency Training Program in Internal Medicine, Diversity Curriculum Taskforce.

the mnemonic RESPECT, that summarizes many of the points discussed in this chapter (see Box 1-3). This model emphasizes several important concepts of the cross-cultural/racial/ethnic communication process. Demonstrating respect is an important first step. Feeling disrespected is a major complaint of many racial and ethnic minority groups and can result in patients making decisions not to return for care. Respect may be shown with an act as simple as calling a black women "Mrs Smith" instead of "Miss Smith" or using her first name only with permission. Knowing whether it is appropriate and how to touch a patient in greeting is another simple way for the physician to be respectful.

Cultural Desire (Internal Motivation)

Cultural competence arises from the desire to improve one's relations with other racial, ethnic, and social groups. Self-awareness of one's own culture, biases, and beliefs is a necessary step in developing cultural competence. A physician asks himself or herself: "Am I doing the best I can to diagnose and treat this patient? How can I improve my relationship with this patient and thus provide better care? Do I have prejudices that affect my diagnoses and treatments?" Self-questioning and internal motivation for positive change are the bases of successful cultural competence.

Summary

Identifying the patient's explanatory model can be accomplished by eliciting the patient's story or perspective of the illness. Performing cultural assessment is key to understanding the patient's perspective. Understanding the pitfalls of the physician/patient power differential is essential to effective communication; this is especially important when working with historically disenfranchised groups. Physicians have sometimes abused their power whether in their recruitment of research subjects or in reporting pregnant women with drug addiction to legal authorities. Fear of how physicians may view them as individuals or of how they will use information that has been shared sometimes leads patients to withhold important information. Displaying empathy is an important aspect of trying to understand the patient's concerns. Eliciting the patient's concerns and emotions is also important to understanding the impact of their circumstances. RESPECT results in the development of a therapeutic alliance with the patient and trust in the physician.

Patients with Limited English Language Proficiency

Legal Issues

Working with patients with limited English language proficiency can be challenging. Communication is more difficult because of the inability of the physician to speak the patient's native language, the inability of the patient to understand the nuances of English, the presence of a third party (i.e., an interpreter) in the doctor/patient relationship, and the lack of supportive administrative structures such as bilingual patient information and education material.

Ethically and legally physicians are required to provide patients with limited English language proficiency with the same standard of care as they do English-speaking patients. Title VI of the Civil Rights Act of 1964 states that "no person in the United States shall on ground of race, color or national origin be excluded from participation and be denied the benefits of or be subjected to discrimination under any program or activity receiving federal financial assistance." This statute covers doctors who treat Medicare or Medicaid patients as well as hospitals that receive federal grants. Under this law doctors cannot employ any practice that has a discriminatory impact on individuals based on their race or national origin. The failure of providers to overcome language barriers may have serious discriminatory effects on non-English-speaking patients, because the latter may be deprived of services that are available to English-speaking patients.

Several practices common in medical settings are legally questionable. These practices include asking non-English-speaking patients to bring their own interpreters to appointments; absence of bilingual or multilingual signs, telephone systems, and patient education materials; and the use of untrained personnel as interpreters.

Why Use a Professional Interpreter?

There are compelling reasons to use interpreters when the patient and physician do not share a common language. Research has demonstrated that patient satisfaction improves and clinical service and receipt of preventive care increase when interpreters are used. Physicians who practice in large groups or in institutions should advocate for trained professional interpreters who are on staff, under contract, or available from interpreter banks, or for access to the ATT language bank.

In general, the use of a family member or friend of the patient as an interpreter should be discouraged because of serious issues of confidentiality, competency in medical interpreting, and the need for physicians to ask sensitive questions related to, for example, domestic violence and sexual behavior. Even if a family member or friend is brought to the office, the physician remains obligated to offer the patient a trained, disinterested interpreter and to have that interpreter speak with the patient to confirm that he or she is declining to use that interpreter in favor of a family member. Explaining that trained interpreters have learned medical terminology and how to interpret in an unbiased way is sometimes helpful. Family members may want to stay as advocates for the patients, and the appropriateness of this should be explored with the patient. Case 1-3 illustrates the pitfalls of using family members as interpreters.

Working with Interpreters

The number and availability of interpreters often depends on the location of the physician's practice. Local, county, and state health departments may track interpreter resources. Hospitals often have interpreter banks and can help to identify someone with specific language skills. Community health centers may also have access to interpreters. Community-based agencies that provide social services to specific minority populations may also be able to locate interpreters, but the physician must make sure that the interpreter has appropriate training and knows medical terminology. The logistics for scheduling an interpreter from one of these sources (i.e., the amount of lead time needed) varies depending on the source. Physicians cannot bill patients for the cost of an interpreter. Some states have financial arrangements that will reimburse providers for the cost and/or pay for interpreter charges for Medicaid patients.

It is not always possible to anticipate that a patient will need an interpreter, but institutions, health plans, and other providers should note this requirement when making a referral. The interpreter should arrive at least ten minutes before the patient's appointment. The doctor should introduce himself to the interpreter and spend a brief period before the patient encounter to understand whether the interpreter is bicultural as well as bilingual. Bicultural interpreters sometimes are able to help explain the cultural context of the interview. For example, an American Indian patient may not advise a physician that it is against his custom to answer questions about

CASE 1-3 A 69-YEAR-OLD CAPE VERDEAN MAN WHO NEEDS AN INTERPRETER

Mr Cesar, a 69-year-old Cape Verdean male who speaks little English, was brought to the emergency department after an attempt to jump off a balcony at a nursing home where he had recently been placed with his wife. He has been evaluated by an internist, but no interpreter was present. His son and daughter-in-law now arrive. His son speaks English well and acts as interpreter for his father when a psychiatrist comes to interview him.

Mr Cesar's son tells the psychiatrist that his father has recently been depressed. Mr Cesar has severe COPD and diabetes and is limited in his activity. He requires assistance with his personal care. Formerly his wife had administered to his needs, but she became disabled after a stroke. When she had to enter the nursing home so did Mr Cesar. The patient did not admit to wanting to jump off the balcony and insisted through his son that he was fine. The psychiatrist suggested possible admission to a psychiatric hospital, but after his discussion with the son agreed that the patient could go back to the nursing home. The psychiatrist recommended that Mr Cesar follow-up with an outpatient psychiatric appointment.

Three days later Mr Cesar was returned to the emergency department after he jumped off a balcony at the nursing home and sustained multiple pelvic fractures.

DISCUSSION

In this situation the patient should have had a complete confidential psychiatric assessment using a trained interpreter. Mr Cesar may not have felt comfortable answering the psychiatrist's questions with his son present. He may have been concerned about the stigma associated with his illness or may not have wanted his son to know how depressed he was. The internist who assessed Mr Cesar should also have insisted on a trained interpreter. Given this patient's co-morbid conditions, the internist should have taken an appropriate history while conducting a complete physical to rule out medical complications or medication reactions that may have contributed to his depressed mood and suicidal behavior.

deceased family members. An interpreter who understands specific American Indian traditions can explain this to the physician and help to devise a strategy to obtain an appropriate family history. The physician should also clarify the role of the interpreter. In some circumstances the interpreter may have a dual role such as patient advocate or medical assistant.

The physician and interpreter should also agree on the type of interpretation to be used: phrased, simultaneous, or summary. With *phrased interpretation* the physician uses short phrases and the interpreter translates as accurately as possible. The physician and interpreter talk in tandem. This generally is the most preferable style of interpreting in a medical situation. With *simultaneous interpretation* the interpreter translates as the physician speaks. This method is often confusing to all three parties involved. With *summary interpretation* the physician and patient make longer statements and the interpreter summarizes what was said.

The interpreter's presence adds significant new dimensions to the doctor/patient interaction. In the ideal situation the physician uses the interpreter as a bridge between himself and the patient. In this context the patient, interpreter, and physician discuss the questions and answers with the hope of reaching a mutual understanding between the former and the latter. If possible, it is helpful for the physician to give the interpreter an overview of the prospective line of approach before meeting with the patient. Inform the interpreter of any time constraints. Tell the interpreter where you want him or her to sit. Ideally the interpreter should sit next to the doctor so that the patient can look at the doctor and interpreter simultaneously. Begin by explaining that all information shared in the interview is confidential and that no one may disclose it without the patient's permission.

The physician should learn some phrases of basic greeting in the patient's native language. This may help to ease discomfort between the doctor and the patient and shows the latter that the former is trying to decrease the barriers to communication. It is important that the physician appear not to be rushed. The physician should maintain the same effort to establish rapport with the patient as he or she would with an English-speaking patient. Skipping inquiries about the patient's family or important events in the patient's life to save time is not recommended. The physician should address the patient directly as opposed to talking to the interpreter and using phrases such as "Ask the patient...."

Ask the patient short questions without complicated clauses. Avoid questions with several parts such as "Have you had chest pain, shortness of breath, or fevers?" and instead ask one question at a time so that the interpreter understands the question and gets the appropriate answer to each. Avoid medical jargon. Keep comments and explanations brief. When lengthy explanations are necessary break them up into small parts.

Some questions may not make sense culturally to the interpreter or patient. For example, asking about time parameters (how long chest pain lasted or what happened weeks before) may seem irrelevant to a patient who is not as time bound as American physicians. Rephrase questions that appear to lead to confusion on the part of the interpreter or the patient.

Summarize what you have heard from the interpreter. Use statements that invite modification: "Correct me if I am wrong, but this is what I understood you to say. . . . Is that correct?" Pursue unconnected issues that the patient raises. These issues may lead to crucial information or uncover new information about the patient. They may also uncover difficulties with the process of interpretation. To better give instructions to patients, provide written materials if available in the patient's native language. If language-appropriate materials are not available, ask the interpreter to write down the important points.

At the end of the session ask the interpreter if he or she had any concerns about the interview. Share your concerns with the interpreter and get any useful clarifying information. If disturbing or difficult issues were discussed, offer some words of support to the interpreter. Providers should document in the patient chart that an interpreter was used to obtain the medical history, the interpreter's name, and the amount of time the interpreter spent with the patient.

In circumstances when an interpreter is not available providers can use the ATT language line services. The services are available 24 hours, 7 days a week, and offer over 140 languages. The interpreters are often native speakers and undergo special training to ensure their skill and accuracy. Providers and institutions may subscribe to this service on a monthly basis. Nonsubscribers may use the service by calling a toll-free number

(1-800-628-8486). The service is expensive, however, costing more than $3 per minute.

Providers who have some experience with a foreign language often try to speak to patients without the use of interpreters. Research demonstrates that providers usually overestimate their language proficiency and patients often do not understand what the provider is communicating. Physicians should always use interpreters unless sure of their multilingual fluency.

Summary

Medicine faces challenging times as the population of the United States becomes increasingly diverse and inequities in health care and disparities in health status are repeatedly documented. Physicians who want to be competent in caring for diverse populations require specific knowledge, attitudes, and skills to be successful in this endeavor. Self-awareness of one's own culture, biases, and beliefs is a necessary step in developing cultural competence. Acknowledging difference, developing effective communication skills, and adapting skills to meet the needs of racial and ethnic groups are necessary. Cultural competence is a means for achieving effective relationships with patients and for ensuring that they receive the highest quality of care.

REFERENCES

1. Polednak AP. Racial and ethnic differences in disease. New York: Oxford University Press; 1989:32.
2. Williams D. Race and health: basic questions, emerging directions. Ann Epidemiol. 1997;7:332-7.
3. US Census Bureau. Census 2000 and 1990 Census of Population, General Population Characteristics (1990 CP-1).
4. Barzansky B, Etzel SI. Education programs in US medical schools, 2000-2001. JAMA. 2001;286:1049-55.
5. Moy E, Bartman BA. Physician race and care of minority and medically indigent patients. JAMA. 1995;273:1515-20.
6. US Department of Health and Human Services. Report of the Secretary's Task Force on Black and Minority Health. Washington, DC: US Government Printing Office; 1985.
7. US Department of Health and Human Services. Healthy People 2010: Understanding and Improving Health; Nov. 2000.
8. Kaiser Family Foundation Survey of Race, Ethnicity and Medical Care: Public Perceptions and Experiences; Oct. 1999.
9. Collins KS, Hall A, Neuhaus C. US Minority Health: A Chartbook. New York: The Commonwealth Fund; 1999.

10. US Department of Health and Human Services. Health, United States, 2000. DHHS: Hyattsville, MD; 2000.

11. Wood AJJ. Racial differences in the response to drugs: pointers to genetic differences. N Engl J Med. 2001;344:1392-6.

12. Canadian Public Health Ministry. Tyler Norris Community Initiatives.

13. Mayberry RM, Mili F, Vaid IGM, et.al. Racial and ethnic differences in access to medical care: a synthesis of the literature. Henry J. Kaiser Family Foundation; 1999.

14. Hall JA, Roter DL, Katz NR. Meta-analysis of correlates of provider behavior in medical encounters. Med Care. 1988;26:657-75.

15. Goldman R, Monroe AD, Dube C. Ann Behav Sci Med Educ. 1996;3:37-46.

16. Pinderhughes E. Understanding Race, Ethnicity and Power: The Key to Efficacy in Clinical Practice. New York: Free Press; 1989.

17. Harwood A. Ethnicity in Medicine. Cambridge, MA: Harvard University Press; 1981.

18. Jones JH. Bad Blood: The Tuskegee Syphilis Experiment—A Tragedy of Race and Medicine. New York: Free Press; 1981.

19. Nichols E. Private communication.

20. Harwood A. Guidelines for culturally appropriate health care. In: Harwood A, ed. Ethnicity and Medical Care. Cambridge, MA: Harvard University Press; 1981:483-507.

21. Berlin EA, Fowkes WC. A teaching framework for cross-cultural health care. West J Med. 1983;139:935.

22. Kleinman A, Eisenberg L, Good B. Culture, illness, and care: clinical lessons from anthropologic and cross-cultural research. Ann Intern Med. 1978;88:251-8.

2

Care of Blacks and African Americans

MELISSA WELCH, MD

The health status of African Americans and other black Americans continues to lag behind that of other racial and ethnic groups (1); this persistent disparity and its contributing factors have been extensively described (2-4). Even with societal consensus on approach and sufficient resources, closing of the black-white health status gap is uncertain (5). Furthermore, the relation between blacks and the medical establishment has been bittersweet (6,7). Although blacks have enjoyed the improved overall survival rates experienced by all races and ethnic groups during the last century (4), they have also suffered morbidity in the name of "medical advancement" (6).

Missed opportunities to establish trust and a therapeutic alliance between providers and African American patients persist. As with any ethnic group, family social structure and influences, geographic distribution, environmental risks, communication patterns, and lifestyle preferences influence the health beliefs and behaviors of African Americans. Generally, however, African Americans still lack overall confidence in the health care system and believe they are less likely to receive the same medications, treatments, or quality of care as whites (8). Providers must meet the challenge of improving African American health outcomes by directly addressing important issues and building a foundation of trust with the black community.

Definitions

African Americans are people of African descent who live in the United States. The term *black* is used in a similar manner; this term is common in the scientific literature. Strictly speaking, *African Americans* are descended from the slaves brought to America during the 18th and 19th centuries, whereas *blacks* in the United States comprise a diversity of ethnicities and cultures including recent large immigrant groups from Africa and the Caribbean. Throughout this chapter the terms are used interchangeably unless otherwise noted.

Demographics and Diversity

According to Census 2000, 36.4 million people, or 12.9% of the total population, reported as being black or African American. The state with the largest number of blacks is New York, but more than half of the blacks in the country live in the South (9). It is predicted that the South will experience the largest growth in black population in the next few decades.

Although there are important similarities among African Americans, the geographic distribution of blacks across the United States highlights the heterogeneity within the population. African American diversity can be mapped by "cultural ecological areas" that vary in history, economics, and social and environmental factors. Some areas, for example, have been influenced by French traditions (Louisiana, eastern coastal Texas, southwestern Mississippi) or American Indian culture (Oklahoma, parts of Arkansas and Kansas); several large cities comprise a group of post-1920 metropolitan ghetto/inner-city areas (New York City, Detroit, Chicago, San Francisco) (10).

Assumptions that African Americans are monolithic in their beliefs and behaviors almost invariably lead to stereotyping, incorrect ideas about ethnicity, lack of understanding of health beliefs, and poor patient compliance. For example, consider a black female naturalized citizen born in Panama, bilingual in English and Spanish, who has health beliefs and behaviors based on Panamanian and Caribbean ancestral influences. The physician who manages her diabetes needs to understand how her dietary patterns may be similar to (couscous, pickled pig's feet), yet different from (fewer fried foods, plantains, raw fish), those of most American-born blacks. The provider must also consider the use of salves, teas, and other home remedies that may be specific to her cultural origin.

Among rural, lower income, and older African Americans, health care providers more frequently find health beliefs and practices based on traditional African healing such as medicinal roots, herbs, and leaves. Most African Americans in urban areas follow popular health care beliefs. Recent immigrants from Africa or the Caribbean who live in urban areas, however, may also assume traditional folk traditions. This "within-group" diversity is one of the most compelling reasons for providers to acknowledge and respect not only the race or ethnicity of a patient but also the culture with which the patient personally identifies. Questioning, not stereotyping, leads to better understanding of the patient and to more successful treatment.

Racial Discrimination and Prejudice

The persistent disparities in health care access and disease morbidity and mortality of African Americans versus whites are not completely understood. *Excess mortality* is mortality that cannot be explained by well-established medical and social risk factors for disease such as smoking or poverty. The question remains open as to which unexplained factors (e.g., race itself or discrimination) account for the excess morbidity observed among blacks. Up to 31% of the excess mortality in African Americans remains unexplained once income and known risk factors for disease are taken into account (3).

Researchers have proposed a physiologic response to racism that may account for the excess prevalence of conditions such as hypertension or low-birth-weight babies among blacks (10,10a,11). Also, national surveys have demonstrated that blacks are less likely than whites to have a usual source of health care (12), so delayed access to care may contribute to the observed increases in disease morbidity and mortality in low-income and minority groups. Examples include the tendency of blacks to use emergency departments when symptoms can no longer be ignored, often late in the course of disease, and the tendency to seek peer, rather than professional, advice about preventive screening such as mammography or HIV testing.

Even when African Americans gain access to health care they are less likely than whites to receive some therapies (13-16). This disturbing trend is not easily explained by risk factor analysis or by studies that simply adjust for race and class effects (17). In examining the poorer health status of blacks one must consider a causal mechanism that takes into account discrimination as a factor regardless of economic status (2). Blacks of all economic levels experience discrimination in health care. Consider the experience of Betty, a 40-year-old black woman who works in health care. Here she describes her experience with a health care provider during a visit for a Pap smear:

I went to this doctor. I had an infection. . . . She said, "How many sex partners do you have?" I said "Gulp" and just looked at her. . . . She said, "Oh, you don't know how many". . . . I felt like I was a little piece of garbage. I was just . . . stereotyped: "There was a little black woman who's out havin' all of these men who comes in here with an infection. . . . " (18)

The Commonwealth Fund reports that blacks commonly experience disrespect in the health care setting (12). Assumptions based on negative societal images of blacks contribute to the negative experiences many blacks encounter when they present for health care. For example, multiple general assumptions are often made about black women's sexual preferences and behaviors. The most common assumption is sexual promiscuity, usually assigned to black women from low-income backgrounds who are also assumed to exchange sex for drugs. Betty's experience of being made to feel inferior when she presented for a routine Pap smear is unfortunately not uncommon: her values, sexual orientation, and risk factors were never elicited. For many blacks, receiving health care is all too often a degrading and humiliating experience. Often insults are subtle but nonetheless perceived by the black patient.

As stated earlier, making assumptions based on a patient's race, ethnicity, or culture impairs culturally competent care. Preferences, risk behaviors, and individual patient experiences must always be confirmed through direct inquiry.

Social and Environmental Risks

Like socioeconomic status, social and environmental risk factors represent significant hazards to the overall health and well-being of African Americans. A significant proportion of blacks live in urban areas plagued by violent crime, in close proximity to toxic waste sites, and in older housing (2,19). These conditions lead to significant mortality.

Violence experienced by many urban blacks has had a major adverse impact on the African American population. Homicide is the leading killer of black men between the ages of 15 and 34 (20). The violence in many inner-city communities is linked to crime that stems from the use of drugs and alcohol (21,22). Resources beyond those available to the primary care provider are necessary to decrease violence in the black community. However, because violence is related to drug use and drug-seeking behavior

(21), recognizing and reducing substance abuse should be a major priority for health care providers. Physicians who have patients with drug and alcohol problems should be assertive about offering access to treatment services.

Diet and Exercise

Poor diet and lack of exercise are modifiable risk factors that provide a good opportunity for provider intervention, which, if successful, can result in reduction of obesity and cardiovascular morbidity (23). Some African American dietary traditions and lifestyle patterns are a challenge to the management of chronic diseases such as hypertension, diabetes, and cardiovascular disease, and to overall weight control.

Many American-born blacks enjoy pork products with high salt content; traditional festive foods including fried chicken and heavy gravies (made from meat drippings) are common. Because African Americans on average have higher-fat, lower-fiber diets than whites, they should be encouraged to adopt alternative diets that maintain cultural traditions where possible (Table 2-1) (24,25). The Web site of the Southeastern Michigan Dietetic Association (www.semda.org) provides a version of the USDA food pyramid for healthy eating that is adapted for African American foods.

Table 2-1 Recommendations for Decreasing Risks Associated with Traditional African American Foods

Traditional Food	Healthy Alternative
Macaroni and cheese	• Use low-fat and reduced-salt cheese • Use 1% or skim milk
Fried chicken	• Oven "fried" chicken • Baked chicken • Barbecue chicken
Potato salad	• Use low-fat mayonnaise • Use olive oil, herb, and mustard dressing
Pound cake	• Angel food cake
Collard greens or green beans with salt pork	• Substitute smoked turkey neck for pork
Barbecue spare ribs	• Limit size of serving and number of helpings

Also important to the physician is an awareness of geographic and intra-group differences and their influence on dietary habits. Blacks who are immigrants (Cuban, West Indian, native Africans), for example, do not have the same food preferences or dietary practices as blacks raised in America. Similarly, the Kosher diets practiced by black Muslims exclude pork or pork products.

Based on self-reported data from national surveys, African Americans are generally described as more sedentary than whites (26), although extensive research on the exercise patterns of African Americans and their influence on health outcomes is lacking.

Gender Roles

Black Women

Female slaves generally worked in the households of their masters. Their "Mammy" image was characterized by the faithful and devoted domestic servant who submitted to her role as such and who, as a slave, received no compensation. Yet, in her own domain, the female slave was the primary caregiver, albeit one often submissive to her male partner.

Conflicting roles persist in the lives of contemporary African American women. Black women are often single heads of households and outnumber black men in the workforce, but they are among the lowest paid workers (27). Consequently they often carry a heavy load of work and home responsibilities. Furthermore, although extended family networks and kinship support systems may provide black women with help for their many duties, these same networks can themselves bring unrelenting obligations.

Stress caused by these burdens crosses economic lines. Coupled with the high incidence of multiple health problems afflicting African American women (Case 2-1), it becomes imperative for providers to find ways to support the attempts of these patients to recognize their own health needs (28).

Black Men

Like African American women, black men have historically suffered role conflicts. Slavery stripped black men of their masculinity, forcing them to be submissive servants, useful solely because of their physical strength. Slavery's tragically negative impact is evident today in the struggle of black men to be respected as intelligent leaders and as wage-earners and supporters of their families.

CASE 2-1 A 37-YEAR-OLD OBESE AFRICAN AMERICAN WOMAN WITH CHRONIC LOW BACK PAIN, MENORRHAGIA, AND HIV INFECTION

Anna Jones is a 37-year-old obese African American woman with chronic low back pain and menorrhagia. Her menorrhagia is secondary to a large uterine myoma. Preoperative analysis of blood for autologous transfusion reveals that she is HIV-infected. She denies previous exposure. She has been married to a new partner for 1 year, and though she states that he is HIV-negative Mrs Jones has no medical proof of this. She is devastated by the news and becomes depressed. Her primary HIV care needs are repeatedly postponed by her own denial and the care of her elderly mother-in-law. She has a daughter with special learning needs who is unaware of her mother's HIV status. The family is plagued by financial problems.

DISCUSSION

For many African American women, especially those from low socioeconomic backgrounds, competing life priorities make it difficult to attend to personal health needs. Consequently, serious illness may only come to a physician's attention after significant morbidity develops.

Mrs Jones epitomizes the black woman whose family needs precede her own. Besides underscoring the importance of HIV prevention, her case serves to remind providers to offer social and culturally specific peer support groups or programs to help the black woman prioritize her own health needs.

Often denied access to traditional avenues that project masculinity (e.g., higher education, well-paying jobs), many black men employ other means to prove their manliness, often through expressive mannerisms and behaviors (29). Certain demeanors, styles of dress or hair, content and flow of speech, and handshakes distinguish black male mannerisms. These adaptive coping strategies may help black men maintain positive feelings about themselves. Many black men have justifiably painful feelings but, because traditional masculine norms do not include displays of emotion, these feelings are often concealed. Attempts to hide painful emotions may include aloof expressions, detached behaviors, fearlessness, or lack of expression.

Within black culture, the black male behaviors and characteristics described here are not viewed as defenses against pain and sadness but as expressions of strength, power, and courage. These forms of communication use an alternative image of masculinity that in turn enhances self-esteem and shields African American men from the harsh societal realities they face every day (29). With the attainment of higher education and economic advantage, black men may exhibit fewer of these behaviors; however, because blacks of all economic levels face similar biased treatment, middle-income black men may at times demonstrate these same alternative masculine behaviors (29).

To establish empathetic and mutually respectful provider-patient interactions, providers caring for black men must appreciate and understand the historical context of black male masculinity. Because some groups of black men (e.g., adolescents and young adults) rarely present to the physician's office for health care, there is an even greater need to express empathy and support to those who do.

Sexual Relationships

Behaviors of a personal nature such as sexual activity are not easily altered without changing other aspects of the personal life. Gender dynamics influence the sexual behaviors of African American men and women. The sex ratio imbalance (the ratio of single adult men to single adult women) is more prominent among African Americans than among whites (75:100 versus 81:100) (30). The significance of the sex-ratio imbalance is important to consider when defining risk reduction strategies for sexually transmitted diseases and AIDS. For example, an African American woman asking a male partner to use a condom may face several risks, including the loss of the relationship or a violent or abusive response (30).

The disclosure of past sexual activity is often not expected in an African American male-female relationship until the relationship is well established. Risk reduction messages advocating that a partner use condoms and maintain monogamy fail when there is the possibility that a partner will lie about having other partners and refuse to use a condom. Because 65% of African American women are unmarried and the ratio of single black women to single black men is high, monogamy on the part of both partners may be an unrealistic expectation (30) but, despite the challenges, urging black women and men to use condoms remains a useful risk reduction strategy. It is encouraging that recent studies suggest that minority women, especially low-income women, are becoming more empowered in their ability to negotiate condom use with their male partners (31).

Black Lesbians, Gay Men, and Bisexual Men and Women

Black lesbian and bisexual women have been rarely studied. It is clear that black lesbians face multiple oppressions: homophobia, sex discrimination, and racism. Their rates of depression are as high as those of HIV-infected men (32) despite the relatively low risk of HIV infection among lesbians. Safe-sex practices must still be encouraged, however, because the risk of other sexually transmitted infection (e.g., chlamydia) is significant.

As with lesbian women, gay and bisexual black men appear to be at higher risk for depressive symptoms (32). Depression among these men is increased in those who are known to be HIV positive or at risk for HIV infection (32). Black gay or bisexual men are fearful of discovery and stigmatization by the black community. Alternatively, they may not consider themselves to be gay or bisexual, depending on the circumstances under which they have sex with men. Many of these men (as well as bisexual women and lesbians) have issues of low self-esteem, internalized homophobia, and confusion about their sexual identity; therefore they may be less likely to seek health care (33).

The stress and anxiety of decreased acceptance by the black community and, sometimes, by family members may increase dysfunctional coping strategies such as alcohol or drug abuse. Providers should refer lesbian, gay, and bisexual men and women with depressive symptoms to culturally specific programs that can connect them with a support network and decrease their isolation (33).

Domestic Violence

Domestic violence remains a concern among the black population. Contradictions experienced in the form of dichotomous images ("submissive" versus "matriarch") and expectations ("strong" yet "self-sacrificing") imposed on black women may put them at risk for domestic violence (34). Among low-income inner-city African American women, poor social support and psychological stress have been linked to partner violence (35), and low-income black women who are victims of violence are also more likely to experience depressive symptoms and a lower perceived health status (36).

Strategies for preventing episodes of domestic violence generally include universal screening in clinical settings, including primary care offices, emergency departments, and urgent care settings. Providers should be aware of the risks women take in reporting abuse: fear of retaliation, family separation, and possible rejection by family and friends for sharing a private family problem with others. Black women may be more reluctant to get restraining orders or to involve the criminal justice system because of the complex relationship between the black community and the police. Primary care physicians should offer referrals to counseling services that can help patients cope with anger and denial and improve interpersonal relationship skills (37).

Family Influences

The African American extended family is an important resource for effective prevention strategies and behavioral change (38). Families are often broadly defined to include extended relationships rooted in the lineage of the father or mother. Unrelated persons identified as being valuable to the family are frequently given titles such as "Aunt", "Uncle", "Brother", or "Sister". These individuals may be called upon to lend support in times of serious illness or death and may be influential in bringing about the behavioral change needed to prevent disease.

Black families have a greater proportion of female-headed households than white families. Because black women are the lowest wage earners among all race/gender groups (27), many black families live at or below the poverty level. During the past decade, because of multiple societal influences, there has also been an increase in the number of households with no parents, in which grandparents are the major caretakers. Single women or grandmothers heading black households may view their own health as a competing, and lesser, priority than the health of their children. Prevention and treatment of acute and chronic medical conditions may therefore be postponed, contributing to delayed diagnosis and higher disease morbidity and mortality.

Elderly Men and Women

Men and women over 75 years of age represent the fastest growing segment of the American population, and by 2050 blacks are projected to have the largest elder population of all American ethnic groups (39). Unfortunately, it is not unusual to see older black patients with multiple major chronic medical problems (cardiovascular disease, diabetes, hypertension, glaucoma, cerebrovascular disease, renal disease) (40). Because many older blacks define health in terms of the ability to complete tasks of daily living (self-care, traveling, shopping), they may delay seeking health care or deny pain and discomfort if they are able to complete these tasks (41). Delays in seeking care together with the increased likelihood of living in a stressful home environment (neighborhood crime, poor environmental conditions) and increased responsibilities for child rearing contribute to significant psychological stress and chronic disease morbidity (42).

Careful history taking (e.g., educational attainment, work history, significant social supports, geographic origin, African ancestry) can facilitate the physician's success in having a trusting relationship with older patients. Understanding the unique lives of black elderly patients also helps providers identify coping abilities and support systems. The black elder's mantra of "making do with the Lord's help" (43) is an indication that providers need to consider traditional African American values of church and family as key support systems for older blacks. Engaging family, friends, and clergy in the care of the elderly black patient can significantly reduce psychological morbidity and may encourage health-seeking behavior (42).

As with all elderly patients, physicians should pay close attention when prescribing multiple medications because of associated adverse reactions. The physician should routinely assess the elder patient's functionality by testing vision and hearing. The need for home care, transportation, and other supports for maintaining the activities of daily living must also be reviewed.

Communication and Language

African American communication styles include direct eye contact, conveying a sense of concern for the person and the problem, a nonjudgmental approach, and listening. African Americans often use eye contact differently than whites: the former tend to look at the listener while speaking but may look away when listening. Giving personal space without appearing cold, insensitive, or discriminatory is critical for the physician. Providers should ask about the patient's preference or seek permission before addressing elderly black patients by their first name.

Avoidance of negative stereotyping and the sober consideration of the individual's opinion is also important when communicating with African Americans. Some blacks believe that whites, in particular, tend to dominate discussions and intellectualize and thus fail to hear or value the opinions of others (44). Health messages that provide instructions and teach skills are more effective than telling blacks what not to do (45).

Asking for clarification from the patient when he or she uses slang is necessary to ensure the communication of important clinical symptoms or to clarify the patient's understanding of prevention or treatment measures. Providers should refrain from using slang themselves to appear "hip" because the patient may be offended and unclear about the provider's intent. A basic knowledge of current slang phrases may be useful, however, when communicating with younger patients.

Besides slang, there are various regional terms used to describe medical conditions. Among immigrants from Haiti, Jamaica, and the Bahamas, and among many southern blacks, for instance, blood may be characterized as *low* or *high*, referring to anemia as opposed to hypertension. *Spells*, also called *falling outs*, are perceived to be a result of *low blood;* elderly blacks especially may refer to *having had a spell. Shock* is a common term for a stroke. Other common terms include *having sugar, sweet blood*, or *thin blood*, referring to diabetes. Understanding the meaning of these terms is necessary to establish a diagnosis and negotiate an agreeable management plan with the black patient.

Health Beliefs and Practices

Despite differences in age groups, geographic distribution, and socioeconomic levels, general similarities are evident among African American health beliefs and practices. Strong social support networks, belief in the well-being of the community, use of informal health care systems for information (46), mistrust of the medical establishment (6), and fears and fatalism related to cancer (47) are common themes. Blacks have long used prayer and religiosity to cope with and treat health concerns and, although blacks necessarily differ in their religious beliefs (Christianity and Islam being only the most prominent), religion and religious institutions fulfill many roles and often provide both spiritual and psychological support (48). Many black women, for example, across all socioeconomic levels, believe in the power of prayer and God's healing power to treat and cope with breast cancer (47). Although praying and "letting God take care of things" is a major emotional support for many African Americans (especially among elderly women), it can often lead to delays in seeking professional health care.

Many low-income blacks traditionally separate illness into two categories (49). *Natural illness* occurs as a result of God's will or when a person comes into unhealthy contact with the forces of nature, such as exposure to cold or impurities in the air, food, or water. Natural illness can also occur as a punishment for sins. Cures for natural illness include an antidote or other logical protective actions. *Unnatural illness,* on the other hand, is considered the result of evil influences that alter God's intended plan. These illnesses are often founded on a belief in witchcraft, in which individuals exist who possess power to mobilize the forces of good and evil. The use of voodoo healers among Haitians and other West Indian blacks is an example. Treatment or cures for unnatural illness can be found in religion, magic, amulets, and herbs. Many of these beliefs are African in origin, and aspects of them may be seen among African Americans of all backgrounds.

Beliefs and practices regarding terminal illness are less well described. Ethiopians and Eritreans generally prefer that the family, rather than the patient, be informed of a terminal illness (50). They have a strong belief in destiny and God's power to influence events, especially health events. Among many West Indian and Central American blacks, communication about an upcoming death or communication with the dead may often be revealed through dreams.

Attempts at spiritual healing may be concealed from providers to avoid the stigma attached to such practices, which may be labeled as devil worshipping or mumbo-jumbo by mainstream European-American culture (50). When such medical or health-related information is revealed, providers should place it in its proper cultural context. Insofar as possible the physician should work with the patient to accommodate personal beliefs into any treatment plan.

Specific Diseases

Diabetes

In 1998 approximately 1.5 million of the 35 million blacks in the United States had been diagnosed with diabetes (51). An estimated additional 730,000 African Americans have diabetes yet do not know they have the disease. Diabetes is two to four times more prevalent in blacks than in whites and is particularly common among middle-aged and older adults and among women. Compared to whites, African Americans with diabetes are more likely to develop complications (end-stage renal disease, retinopathy, and limb amputations) and to experience greater disability as a result. The diabetes mortality rate is 27% higher among blacks than whites (51).

Type 2 diabetes is the most common among African Americans. It is caused by impaired insulin secretion and resistance to the action of insulin. Major medical risk factors for Type 2 diabetes among blacks include obesity, higher levels of fasting insulin (hyperinsulinemia), gestational diabetes, and lack of physical activity (23,51). Among these risks, obesity is the most significant, and there is a disproportionate number of African Americans with both diabetes and obesity (23). Obesity is thought to play a causal role in 50% to 90% of non-insulin-dependent diabetes cases (23).

Prevention and education are central to reducing diabetes morbidity and mortality among blacks. Increased awareness of the disease must be raised in the black community through acceptable venues such as faith-based institutions. Emphasis on the importance of control of glucose levels to prevent early complications among patients already diagnosed with diabetes must be stressed, as well as the importance of increased physical activity and healthy dietary choices. Culturally sensitive education of risks and alternative diet plans must be consistently reinforced by the clinician. African American women respond to group activities that reinforce exercise and dietary changes.

Obesity in Women

African American women have higher rates of obesity than men and other racial groups (23). Among African American women, obesity-related morbidity includes diabetes (relative risk = 2.5 deaths per 100,000 compared to whites), osteoarthritis (two times the age-specific incidence versus whites 25 to 34 years old), hypertension (18% attributed to obesity), altered lipid profiles (elevated LDL), and cancers and benign tumors such as uterine fibroids (23,52).

Traditional weight management programs may not be effective with black women. Being overweight is often the norm in black female peer groups, and low self-esteem is not observed among overweight and obese black female adolescents or women. Overweight African American women are also less likely to feel guilty about overeating, less likely to consider themselves overweight, and 2.5 times less likely to be dissatisfied with their weight than whites (53). There is evidence from national weight loss intervention surveys that blacks lose less weight on average than whites (52), but when black women do perceive themselves to be overweight they are as likely as whites to attempt weight loss (54). African American tolerance for obesity may lessen their motivation for weight loss attempts (55), so strategies for weight management must be culturally sensitive and individualized (Box 2-1).

Cardiovascular Disease

Vascular disease, including stroke, coronary artery disease, and hypertension, are significant contributors to the differential mortality rates between blacks and whites (23). Coronary heart disease mortality is the single largest killer of men and women. Age-adjusted prevalence of coronary heart disease among adults over the age of 20 is 7.1 times higher for black men and 9 times higher for black women than for white men and women, respectively. Hypertension in African Americans occurs earlier than in whites and is more severe (23). As a result of earlier and more severe hypertension, blacks have a 1.3

Box 2-1   Suggestions for Managing Obesity in African Americans

- Provide information about serious health conditions associated with being overweight and obese.
- Promote weight control as a means of achieving increased self-esteem.
- Recognize that perceptions of obesity may be different in the black community.
- Offer weight loss programs that are individualized and sensitive to food preferences.
- Assess client preparedness and motivation by using the Prochaska/DiClemente Stages of Change Model.
- Assess for eating binges by inquiring about unresolved stress and other illness.
- Encourage realistic expectations and milestones.
- Emphasize the need to incorporate exercise into daily patterns of activity (e.g., doing housework, playing with children, using stairs instead of elevators); emphasize fitness over thinness.
- Encourage communal exercise (e.g., group walks) and emotional support through peer groups or "Sister Circles."
- Ask about dinners after 8:00 P.M. and late-night snacking.
- Recommend alternatives to alcohol or "lighter" alcoholic beverages.

---

times greater risk of nonfatal stroke, 1.5 times greater risk of heart disease death, and 4.2 times greater rate of end-stage kidney disease than whites (23). African American men and women have a two- to three-fold greater risk of ischemic stroke than whites and are more likely to die of stroke (23).

Increased risk factors for cardiovascular disease in blacks include hypertension, obesity, diabetes, cigarette smoking, elevated cholesterol, physical inactivity, and delayed diagnosis caused by delays in seeking care. Targeted strategies to educate and engage patients in risk reduction efforts are critical. In a survey of opinions on the causes of common medical conditions, older blacks were three times more likely to attribute heart disease and hypertension to stress and overwork (56,57). Similarly, blacks may report fewer painful symptoms and attribute cardiac symptoms to noncardiac origins, resulting in delays in care seeking (58). These findings underscore the importance of understanding patient beliefs about the cause of disease and of educating all African American patients about cardiovascular symptoms and risks.

Many recent studies have found that when blacks do present with cardiac symptoms they are less likely than whites to be referred for cardiac diagnostic and treatment procedures, a difference not explained by insurance or patient preference. Blacks are also less likely than whites to be prescribed beta-blockers after a myocardial infarction, but they do appear to respond to cardiac medications differently than whites. Blacks with hypertension demonstrate better reduction in blood pressure when diuretics are used alone or in combination with other drugs. Blacks do not exhibit the same response to ACE-inhibitors (ACE-I) in terms of blood pressure response or congestive heart failure mortality reduction. The differences appear to be due to differences in dietary sodium and different polymorphic genes. It is important to remember, however, that blacks benefit from ACE-I with appropriate doses.

Cancer

Prostate Cancer

Other than superficial skin cancer, prostate cancer is the most frequently diagnosed malignancy; it is the second leading cause of death in American men. The highest incidence of prostate cancer and the greatest mortality is seen in black men, with 5-year survival rates of 90% for whites and 75% for blacks (59). Prevention, early detection, and treatment of prostate cancer in African American men is adversely affected by low socioeconomic status, distrust of the health care system, and delayed presentation, all of which are consistent with the overall discrepancy in black health care (60). Recent evidence offers hope that better access to care and earlier detection and treatment can lead to better outcomes for black men (61,62).

With the advent of the prostate-specific antigen (PSA) screening test, earlier detection of prostate cancer is possible (63). Because of the greater disease risk and the higher incidence of prostate cancer in young black men, some experts recommend PSA screening beginning at 40 to 45 years of age (64). Attention to age-adjusted reference ranges (Walter Reed PSA Reference Range) for PSA is important for maximal cancer detection in all men (63,64). A thorough digital rectal examination is still a recommended adjunct to PSA testing (65).

Breast Cancer

The overall incidence of breast cancer is highest among white women, although mortality rates are higher in African American women (66). Black women present with more advanced stages of breast cancer than white women.

Among young women (younger than 40 years), breast cancer rates are higher in blacks than in whites. This crossover in the age-specific incidence of breast cancer between the two races has existed since 1969 (67). Differences in breast cancer risks by age and class groupings within and across ethnic groups (67) suggest a positive association between higher social class and higher breast cancer risk among young black women. In contrast, no relation between social class and breast cancer risk has been observed among young white women. Whether social class alone can explain the increased breast cancer risk in young black women is uncertain. Higher average body mass index and increased levels of estrogen have also been suggested. Prudent education about the increased risks of breast cancer for young black women is warranted, although whether this will translate into altered screening strategies for mammography or breast self-examination requires additional research.

Counseling black women of any age about breast cancer prevention is critical to reducing their higher overall breast cancer mortality versus whites. For many black women (young and old) cancer still represents a death sentence (47), and fear of finding out the truth can delay a woman's participation in screening or seeking treatment. Discussions about breast cancer occur infrequently among black women, even when it has afflicted female relatives (47). The spiritual and religious inclination of African

Americans may also adversely influence breast cancer screening behaviors, with women believing screening is futile in the face of god's will (47) or believing that "Jesus will fix it after awhile" (48).

Use of black role models or cancer survivors to promote breast cancer screening and to challenge the notion of cancer as a death sentence are effective for screening and promotion of breast health in black women (68). For example, "breast health parties" fashioned after Tupperware parties and programs that provide escorts to screening centers have been effective in increasing the number of mammograms in both rural and urban settings.

Providers should learn about black women's perceptions of the causes of breast cancer (spider bites, breast feeding, wearing a bra too tight, not wearing a bra) and develop effective educational messages that incorporate these perceptions of the disease. Treatment strategies for black women facing a mastectomy, lumpectomy, or chemotherapeutic treatment must be approached with sensitivity and attention to body image (69). For the young heterosexual black woman, an altered body image may be particularly stressful because of less favorable odds of finding a black male partner (Case 2-2).

Colorectal and Lung Cancer

Colorectal and lung cancer continue to cause significant morbidity and mortality among men and women of all ethnic backgrounds. African American women are more likely to die of cancer of the breast, colon, or rectum than women of any other group, and they have approximately the same mortality from lung cancer as white women. African American men have the highest cancer mortality rates from colon, rectal, lung, and prostate cancer (66).

Both lung and colon cancer are preventable, yet much of the higher cancer morbidity and mortality seen in blacks is due to the late stage of presentation. Decreased access limits participation in early cancer prevention and treatment programs (70). The approach to reducing cancer mortality in African Americans must include increasing prevention and facilitating earlier presentation when malignancies are suspected (66).

In the case of lung cancer the provider must deliver emphatic messages to alter risk behaviors (e.g., smoking), and nicotine gum and smoking cessation programs must be encouraged. Like other smokers, blacks tend to smoke for the immediate relief provided and to cope with stress. Strategies to reduce smoking must be linked to consequences in the here-and-now, to

---

CASE 2-2 A 31-YEAR-OLD AFRICAN AMERICAN WOMAN WITH BREAST CANCER

Beverly Sampson is a 31-year-old African American woman referred for a left breast biopsy after a screening mammography reveals suspicious calcifications. The biopsy reveals breast cancer. Miss Sampson, a computer programmer, is unfamiliar with breast cancer treatment options and is afraid of chemotherapy and of losing her ability to conceive children. She has an aunt who has undergone a mastectomy, and she confides to her physician that she has significant concerns about how her body image may change.

DISCUSSION

To many blacks and other minorities, the diagnosis of cancer represents a virtual death sentence. For the single young black woman faced with breast cancer, besides the fear of approaching death, there is often increased anxiety about finding a mate. Changes to one's body resulting from mastectomy and chemotherapy are seen as unattractive and off-putting. Sterility can be another concern. Cancer, it is often felt, is a sentence to a single (and almost certainly brief) life.

Physicians must also recognize the silence surrounding breast cancer among many black women. Although Miss Sampson was aware of her aunt's diagnosis, little open discussion on the topic occurred within her family. This patient requires a lot of information on her disease.

This case is also useful as a reminder to physicians of the (unexplained) increased prevalence of breast cancer among young affluent African American women. The support of other female black cancer survivors and sensitive counseling on the various treatment options are important strategies in the management of this patient's breast cancer.

---

effects of smoking on other family members, and to the well-being of the community. Because middle-aged and older blacks and low-income women over the age of 35 are more likely to continue to smoke or to initiate smoking at a later age (71,72), physicians should consider these groups at high-risk for lung cancer.

Screening for Cancer

Because blacks may not willingly accept their risk of cancer, multiple education messages by physicians and health educators promoting early cancer screening and detection (e.g., fecal occult blood testing and sigmoidoscopy or colonoscopy for colorectal cancer) are important. Health education programs with connections to community-based efforts are most effective. Physicians must also be mindful of the sensitive nature of certain screening tests (e.g., digital rectal examination, breast and pelvic examinations). Asking for permission to touch the patient and having a heightened sense of respect for the individual are important and increase the likelihood of the patient's return for future periodic screening (73).

Uterine Fibroids

Uterine leiomyomas, commonly known as fibroids, are present in 20% to 25% of reproductive-age women. Fibroids are three to nine times more common in black women than in white women, are commonly multiple, and may weigh up to 100 lb. Malignant transformation is rare, but excessive bleeding occurs in approximately 30% of patients.

Menorrhagia associated with fibroids is the most common indication for hysterectomy in the United States. Among women who have hysterectomies, 65% of black women have fibroids compared with 28% of white women (74). Black women having hysterectomies have more medical and surgical complications (odds ratio = 1.4) and higher mortalities (odds ratio = 3.1) than white women after adjusting for multiple factors (age, co-morbidity, diagnosis, route of surgery, hospital characteristics, and source of payment) (74).

Because black women often have a higher prevalence of obesity (making pelvic assessment for fibroids more difficult) and because they often access care late or when symptoms are already severe, they may present at a stage at which surgical management is the only option (74). Because of previous reproductive abuses by the health care system, black women are often skeptical of the need for, and consequences of, surgery. They therefore often seek nonsurgical interventions such as dietary treatment, herbal treatments, and stress reduction. These methods of treatment have been described in many popular articles and books (34).

Better and wider education on the risk and prevalence of fibroids is needed. Additionally, clinicians should be aware of the higher prevalence of fibroids among black women and screen for them by history and clinical examination. Earlier recognition and management of fibroids can prevent significant excess morbidity and mortality in African American women during the reproductive years.

HIV/AIDS

AIDS disproportionately affects the African American community, and the number of cases continues to grow. For every 100,000 African Americans in 1996, there were 89.7 cases of AIDS reported (75). AIDS continues to be the leading cause of death for African Americans between the ages of 25 and 44 years, with mortality rates for black men four times that of white men and for black women nine times those of white women (75).

Injection drug use remains the most common route of HIV infection among African Americans. Approximately 55% of black women and 42% of black men with AIDS are injection drug users. Of the 34% of AIDS cases that result from sexual contact between heterosexuals, 59% of such cases in women are the result of being the partner of an injection drug user. In 12% to 16% of cases of HIV, the cause is unknown.

Black gay and bisexual men are increasingly at risk for HIV infection (76). They are less knowledgeable about HIV risk behaviors, less revealing about their sexual orientation, more likely to have had female sexual partners, and more likely to use drugs in association with sex than white men who have sex with men (77).

Many minority women are aware of the risk of AIDS but do not personalize that risk. The realities of poverty and of being an ethnic minority are more immediate and pressing than possible HIV infection (30). Many African American (and Latino) women view AIDS as a minor concern compared with obtaining adequate food and shelter, dealing with government agencies and paperwork, and ensuring personal and family safety (see Case 2-1). Even if women wanted to reduce their risks, many may lack the financial resources to do so (30).

Several beliefs held by many low- and middle-income African Americans may impede acceptance of AIDS risk reduction messages: the affirmation of manhood and womanhood through childbearing, the myth of black sexual superiority, and the tendency to exaggerate and give words multiple meanings within a sexual context (78). Manhood/womanhood affirmation is often given as a reason for not using condoms. The myth of black sexual superiority is one that has been carried over to society at large and even more unfortunately is believed by many African Americans. These two beliefs can act in synchrony to reinforce one another. Lastly, in contemporary black culture, talk about sexual activity is often explicit, in loud, colorful language intended to elicit a negative reaction from those unfamiliar with the culture. Individuals skilled in propagating this oral tradition may be held in high regard (78).

The physician should sensitively assess an African American patient's knowledge of AIDS and correct any misconceptions. Many patients may hesitate to ask questions for fear of being labeled ignorant. The physician should make every attempt to get intravenous drug users into multidisciplinary treatment programs as a first step to intervening in the acquisition or spread of HIV infection. Multidisciplinary programs must emphasize family therapy, parenting skills training, life skills training, and adult basic education. Harm reduction through use of needle-exchange programs should also be encouraged for patients who do not choose or fail to achieve abstinence from drugs.

Recognizing that the gender-ratio imbalance may place single African American women in multiple relationships over shorter time periods, physicians should emphasize abstinence, pre-relationship HIV testing, and condom use. More minority women are negotiating condom use by appealing to their partner's sense of responsibility to the family (31). Men and women who are practicing unsafe sex or have more than one partner should also be tested for syphilis, chlamydia, and gonorrhea.

Referral to minority-specific or, preferably, black-specific AIDS service organizations is preferred. A facility that treats mostly white homosexual patients is not the best option for a black patient who may be the only injection drug user, the only woman, or the only African American (33).

Other Sexually Transmitted Infections

Gonorrhea and syphilis rates among the black population continue to exceed those of whites and other ethnic groups. The rapid rise in cases of syphilis during the 1989-90 period may be related to the use of crack cocaine, especially among sexually active adolescents who exchange sex for drugs (79). Although syphilis rates are declining among African Americans, the higher race-specific incidence of syphilis is of concern because syphilis is thought to be a co-vector for HIV infection (80).

Alcohol and Drug Abuse

Alcohol and drug abuse continue to adversely affect the lives of African Americans. According to the National Household Survey on Drug Abuse 2000, blacks and whites use drugs at the same rate (6.4%), but there are disproportionate consequences among African Americans. The high incarceration rate of black men (who comprise almost half of the total prison population) is partly attributable to easily accessible drugs and alcohol in African American communities (81). Lack of alcohol and drug treatment centers in the black community may also be a contributing factor.

Risk Factors

Factors associated with excessive drinking may not apply uniformly to all African American communities, but the general trends are noteworthy. The easy availability of alcohol in black communities and the social use of alcohol for celebrations inadvertently legitimize its use (82). Factors associated with maintaining drinking patterns may also contribute to the increase in illicit drug use (82). Recreational drugs, as well as alcohol, may often be used to cope with personal stress, family problems, and racial tension, and to improve mental functioning (83).

A major factor in drug use is poverty (81). African Americans constitute approximately 10% of the 17.5 million female drug abusers. More than 19% of the women who are admitted to federally funded alcohol and drug treatment programs are poor, and 19% are nonwhite. Among black men, low-income status is a trigger for drug use and trafficking. Drug dealing may be perceived by some as an opportunity to provide for their families and to achieve respect and status (21). However, blacks are not exempt from the growing rates of substance abuse and drug dependency seen among professionals (especially in the health, dental, and legal fields).

Recognition of personal life trauma and psychiatric co-morbidity is central to combating substance abuse among black women. Observational studies suggest that previous sexual abuse, parental substance abuse (and/or a family history of drug or alcohol abuse), and depression are also antecedents to illicit drug use (84,85). Most studies suggest high co-morbidity between psychiatric conditions, sexual abuse, and substance abuse. In a survey of 105 substance-abusing African American women, 61% reported at least one sexual abuse experience. Sixty percent of those identified the perpetrator to be a male family member, more than 60% experienced their first abusive episode before the age of 17 years, and 74% reported three or more depressive symptoms lasting for more than 2 weeks (84). Racism and the experiences of oppression and injustice may also contribute to depression and anger and consequent drug or alcohol abuse.

An African American addicted to drugs suffers from the same biopsychosocial disease as any other addicted person. Its biopsychosocial nature suggests that addiction involves physical brain disease (cravings) complicated by psychosocial factors (emotional triggers, addictive lifestyles, and absence of sober role models). Recovery from addiction therefore involves drug abstinence, which results in the physical and psychosocial changes that support sober living (82,86,87).

Although many of the antecedents to drug addiction are not unique to African Americans, drug abuse among blacks is less often thought of as a disease than as a social problem. Media images of blacks as illicit drug users and of drug-related violence among blacks are misleading and propagate unfortunate stereotypes. Data on drug use contradict such images: whites use illegal drugs at least as much as blacks (81). Drug addiction among blacks must be kept in context and addressed as a medical illness, a disease of addiction, for which medical treatment is necessary. Although the disease of addiction is not race-specific or a respecter of race, social and cultural factors heavily influence recovery and relapse patterns.

Intervention Strategies

Treatment approaches and counseling must be sensitive to cultural issues and incorporate an understanding of the antecedents and factors that contribute to and maintain alcohol and other substance addictions among African Americans. During routine clinical visits, unfortunately, there is little time to intervene in the drug addiction of a patient, and follow-up visits are a necessity.

Specific interventions for treating alcohol and drug abuse in black patients should be part of providing culturally competent outpatient care (Box 2-2). Drug relapses among African Americans recovering from addiction often center on the impact of racial issues such as self-esteem, trust, and self-image. These relapse triggers underscore the importance of recognizing and addressing racism in the treatment program. Establishing a spiritual program, addressing feelings of shame and anger, offering culturally specific peer group support and counseling, providing life skills training and psychiatric

---

Box 2-2   Culturally Competent Outpatient Treatment for Alcohol and Drug Abuse in African Americans

- Avoid assumptions based on race and socioeconomic status.
- Advocate for special services such as life-skill training and culturally specific peer groups.
- Be aware of feelings of shame, guilt, and anger.
- Look for referral programs where patients are of similar background.
- Be sensitive to spiritual issues and incorporate spirituality in the recovery program.
- Offer assistance for previous life trauma (e.g., sexual abuse, harsh experiences of racism).
- Encourage positive self-statements.
- Work toward long-term resolution of the addiction.
- Learn culturally specific relapse triggers and help the patient to avoid them.

---

care, and focusing on individual goals for sobriety and recovery are essential parts of African American recovery programs (86).

Summary

Disparities in the health of blacks compared with whites are linked to multiple factors. Overcoming these disparities will require the collective effort of patients, providers, policy makers, and leaders of the black community. The overall distrust by blacks of physicians and the health care system stems from fears of being unwitting subjects of medical experiments, often in public clinics or hospitals. The Tuskegee Syphilis Study is a prime example (6). Additionally, there exist beliefs that AIDS and the promotion of birth control, for example, are forms of "black genocide" (88).

Despite the challenges, providers can succeed in overcoming distrust and suspicion in the clinical encounter. Cultural sensitivity, including awareness, acceptance, and understanding of the patient's view of his or her illness; an openness to alternative management strategies; and a willingness to hear the patient's story are imperative. Blacks seek the same components of caregiving from physicians that other patients seek: kindness, sympathy, respect, an earnest attempt to assess their ailments, explanations in basic terms, and a shared approach to management. These efforts combined with a genuine expression of interest in the individual as a person, a smile, and a warm tone are universal approaches to patient care that can establish the basis of a lasting and trusting relationship.

Summary of Communication Issues in Caring for African Americans

- Be attentive and listen.
- Be aware of sensitivity towards perceived or actual dismissive attitudes.
- Avoid assumptions about health risk behaviors.
- Ask about specific risks.
- Acknowledge and respect the patient's opinion.
- Give personal space without appearing cold or insensitive.
- Address elders by their surname (Mr/Miss/Mrs).

Summary of High-Risk Diseases and Conditions in African Americans

Be alert for presenting signs of the following diseases and conditions. Keep in mind that history taking needs to consider cultural differences that may otherwise mislead the physician (e.g., reluctance to talk about sexual activity).

Cancer

Breast cancer
- Black women present with more advanced breast cancer.
- Black women do not tend to discuss breast cancer.
- Fear of breast cancer diagnosis and belief that it is a "death sentence" prevent many black women from participating in screening, seeking a diagnosis, or engaging in treatment.
- More diligence is required in counseling black women in a culturally appropriate manner about breast cancer screening.

Colon, rectal, and lung cancer
- Black men have highest mortality rates.
- Blacks tend to present with late-stage disease.

Prostate cancer
- Black men have highest incidence and mortality.
- Screening with PSA beginning in the 40's may be warranted.

(Cont'd.)

Diabetes
- Diabetes is two to four times more prevalent among blacks than whites.
- End-stage consequences of diabetes are more prevalent and severe among blacks.
- Focus on prevention and education (e.g., physical activity, healthy diet choices, control of glucose levels).
- Group activities may be particularly effective.

HIV/AIDS
- Stress importance of condom use.
- Black women may have difficulty negotiating condom use with partner.

Obesity
- Thinness is not valued by blacks as much as by whites; being overweight but fit is acceptable.
- Dietary traditions include foods with high fat and salt content.
- Black women are less likely to report regular physical activity.
- Emphasize disease prevention (diabetes, cardiovascular disease) as objective for weight loss.
- Offer alternative diet plans that maintain culture.
- Peer support programs may be more effective.

Substance Abuse
- Although the overall drug use rate for blacks is the same as for whites, morbidity and mortality are higher for blacks.
- Treatment must be sensitive to unique circumstances of blacks (e.g., higher prevalence of drugs and alcohol in community, increased stress).
- Culturally specific peer group support is important.

Uterine Fibroids
- Uterine fibroids are three to nine times more prevalent in black women.
- Black women have higher rates of hysterectomies.

Cardiovascular Disease
- Hypertension occurs earlier and is more severe in blacks.
- Blacks have a greater risk of end-stage renal disease.
- Blacks may have different responses to cardiovascular drugs (e.g., less responsive to ACE inhibitors).
- Historically, blacks are less likely to be offered invasive cardiac procedures or treatment; blacks are also less likely to be treated with beta-blockers after myocardial infarction.

Violence
- Homicide is the leading cause of death among black men aged 14 to 34.
- Violence is associated with drugs and alcohol.

Summary of Obstacles to Health Care Delivery for African Americans

- Mistrust of medical community.
- Perceived and real bias and disrespect by medical community.
- Black men are less likely to use health care on a regular basis.
- Black women are less likely to have the time and energy for their own health needs due to family responsibilities and other stressors.
- Elderly men and women delay seeking care until activities of daily living are affected.
- Use of alternative interventions for symptoms.
- May be skeptical of cancer screening because of fear of diagnosis and fatalistic attitudes.
- Religious beliefs may lead to a feeling that medical treatment is unnecessary or against God's will.

REFERENCES

1. Projected Life Expectancy at Birth by Race and Hispanic Origin, 1999-2000. 2000 National Projections Program; Washington, DC: Bureau of the Census, Population Division.
2. Cooper R. Health and the social status of blacks in the United States. Ann Epidemiol. 1993;3:137-44.
3. Otten M, Teutsh SM, Williams DF, Mark JS. The effect of known risk factors on the excess mortality of black adults in the United States. JAMA. 1990;263:845-50.
4. Heckler MM. Report of the Secretary's Task Force on Black and Minority Health: Washington, DC: US Government Printing Office; 1985.
5. Nickens H. The role of care, ethnicity, and social class in minority health status. Health Serv Res. 1995;30:151-62.
6. Baker R. Minority distrust of medicine: a historical perspective. Mt Sinai J Med. 1999; 66:212-22.
7. Smith C. African Americans and the medical establishment. Mt Sinai J Med. 1999;66: 280-1.
8. Henry J. Kaiser Family Foundation. Race, Ethnicity and Medical Care: A Survey of Public Perceptions and Experiences. Menlo Park, CA: Henry J. Kaiser Family Foundation; 1999.
9. Campbell P. Population Projections for States by Age, Sex, Race and Hispanic Origin: 1995-2025. Washington, DC: Bureau of the Census, Population Division; 1996.
10. Green V. The black extended family in the United States: some research questions. In: Shinkin D, Shinkin E, Frate E, eds. The Extended Family in Black Society. The Hague: Mouton Degrutor; 1978;378-87.
10a. Krieger N. Racial and gender discrimination: risk factors for high blood pressure? Soc Sci Med. 1990;30:1273-81.
11. Jackson JS, Brown TN, Williams DR, et al. Racism and the physical and mental health status of African Americans: a thirteen year national panel study. Ethn Dis. 1996;6:132-47.

12. Collins KS, Hughes DL, Doty MM, et al. Diverse communities, common concerns: assessing health care quality for minority Americans. Findings from the Commonwealth Fund 2001 Health Care Quality Survey. New York; 2002.

13. Schneider EC, Zaslavsky A, Epstein AM. Racial disparities in quality care for enrollees in Medicare managed care. JAMA. 2002;101:288-94.

14. Bach P, Cramer LD, Warren JL, Begg CB. Racial differences in the treatment of early-stage cancer. N Engl J Med. 1999;34:1198-1205.

15. Guadagnoli E, Ayanian JZ, Gibbons G, et al. The influence of race on the use of surgical procedures for treatment of peripheral vascular disease of the lower extremity. Arch Surg. 1995;130:381-6.

16. Ayanian JZ, Weissman JS, Chasan-Taber S, Epstein AM. Quality of care by race and gender for congestive heart failure and pneumonia. Med Care. 1999;37:1260-9.

17. Pappas G, Queen S, Hadden W, Fisher G. The increasing disparity in mortality between socioeconomic groups in the United States: 1960-1986. N Engl J Med. 1993;329:103-9.

18. Welch M. Race and Socioeconomic Discrimination: Risks for Biased Care. African American Women's Focus Group. Unpublished data; 1996.

19. Johnson R, Coulberson S. Environmental epidemiologic issues and minority health. Ann Epidemiol. 1993;3:175-80.

20. Center for Disease Control and Prevention. Homicide among young black males: United States, 1978-1987. MMWR. 1990;39:869-73.

21. Whitehead TL, Peterson J, Kaljee M. The "hustle": socioeconomic deprivation, urban drug trafficking, and low-income African American male gender identity. Pediatrics. 1994;93:1050-4.

22. Stanton B, Galbrath J. Drug trafficking among African American early adolescents: prevalence, consequences, and associated behaviors and beliefs. Pediatrics. 1994;93(suppl): 1039-43.

23. 2000 Heart and Stroke Statistical Update. Dallas: American Heart Association.

24. Pleas J. Long-term effects of a lifestyle-change obesity treatment program with minorities. J Natl Med Assoc. 1988;80:747-52.

25. Kanders B, Ullman-Joy P, Poreyt JP, et al. The Black American Lifestyle Intervention (BALI): the design of a weight loss program for working-class African American women. J Am Diet Assoc. 1994;943:310-2.

26. National Health and Nutrition Examination Survey III (1988-1994). Bethesda, MD: Centers for Disease Control and Prevention; 1991.

27. Bennet C. The Black Population in the United States: 1993-1994. Washington, DC: Bureau of the Census.

28. Braxton G. Well-being is our birthright: the meaning of empowerment for women of color. Health/PAC Bulletin. Winter 1991:9-11.

29. Harris S. Black male masculinity and same sex friendships. West J Black Studies. 1992;16:74-81.

30. Mays V, Cochran S. Issues in the perception of AIDS risk and risk reduction activities by black and Hispanic/Latino women. Am Psychol. 1988;949-57.

31. Kline A, Kline E, Oken E. Minority women and sexual choice in the age of AIDS. Soc Sci Med. 1992;34:447-57.

32. Cochran S, Mays V. Depressive distress among homosexually active African American men and women. Am J Psychiatry. 1994;151:524-9.

33. Bing E, Soto T. Treatment issues for African Americans and Hispanics with AIDS. Psychiatr Med. 1991;9:455-67.

34. White E. The Black Women's Health Book: Speaking for Ourselves. Seattle: Seal Press; 1994.
35. Thompson MP, Kaslow NJ, Kingree JB, et al. Partner violence, social support, and distress among inner-city African American women. Am J Community Psychol. 2000;28:127-43.
36. Russo NF, Denious JE, Keita GP, Koss MP. Intimate violence and black women's health. Womens Health. 1997;3:315-48.
37. Dennis RE, Key LJ, Kirk AL, Smith A. Addressing domestic violence in the African American community. J Health Care Poor Underserved. 1995;6:284-93.
38. Staples R. The Black Family: Essays and Studies, 5th ed. Belmont, CA: Wadsworth Publishing; 1994.
39. Projections of the United States by Age, Sex, Race and Hispanic Origin: 1992-2050. Washington, DC: Bureau of the Census; 1992.
40. Bernard M. The health status of African American elderly. J Natl Med Assoc. 1993;85:521-8.
41. Harper M. Elderly issues in the African American community. In: Braithwaite R, ed. Health Issues in the Black Community. San Francisco: Jossey-Bass; 1992.
42. Baker F. Psychiatric treatment of older African Americans. Hosp Community Psychiatry. 1994;45:32-7.
43. Franklin A, Jackson J. Factors contributing to positive mental health among black Americans. In: Ruiz D, ed. Handbook of Mental Health and Mental Disorder Among Black Americans. New York: Greenwood; 1990.
44. Ribeau SA, Baldwin JR, Hecht ML. An African-American communication perspective. In Samovar LA, Porter RE, eds. Intercultural Communication: A Reader. Belmont, CA: Wadsworth Publishing; 1994.
45. McClaren P, Juzang I. Reaching the hip-hop generation. Focus: A Guide to AIDS Research and Counseling. 1993;8:1-4.
46. Neighbors H, Jackson J. The use of informal and formal help: four patterns of illness behaviors in the black community. Am J Community Psychol. 1984;12:629-44.
47. Phillips J, Cohen M, Moses G. Breast cancer screening and African American women: "fear, fatalism, and silence." Oncol Nurs Forum. 1999;26:561-71.
48. Abrums M. "Jesus will fix it after awhile": meanings and health. Soc Sci Med. 1999;50:89-105.
49. Snow L. Traditional health beliefs and practices among lower class black Americans. West J Med. 1983;139:820-8.
50. Lipson J, Dibble S, Minark P. Culture and Nursing Care: A Pocket Guide. San Francisco: UCSF School of Nursing Press; 1996.
51. Diabetes in African Americans, 1998. Bethesda, MD: National Institutes of Health.
52. Kumanyika S. Obesity in black women. Epidemiol Rev. 1987;9:31-50.
53. Stevens J, Kumanyika S, Keil J. Attitudes toward body size and dieting: differences between elderly black and white women. Am J Public Health. 1994;84:1322-5.
54. Dawson D. Ethnic differences in female overweight: data from the 1985 National Health Interview Survey. Am J Public Health. 1988;7819:1326-9.
55. Kumanyika S, Morssink C, Agurs T. Models for dietary weight change in African American women: identifying cultural components. Ethn Dis. 1992;2:166-75.
56. Goodwin J, Black S, Shiva S. Aging versus disease: the opinions of older black, Hispanic, and non-Hispanic white Americans about the cause and treatment of medical conditions. J Am Geriatr Soc. 1999;47:973-9.

57. Ontiveros J, Black S, Jakobi P. Ethnic variations in attitudes toward hypertension in adults ages 75 and older. Prev Med. 1999;29:443-9.
58. Raczynski JM, Taylor H, Cutter G, et al. Diagnosis, symptoms, and attribution of symptoms among black and white inpatients admitted for coronary heart disease. Am J Public Health. 1994;84:951-6.
59. Haas GP, Sakr WA. Epidemiology of prostate cancer. CA Cancer J Clin. 1997;47:273-87.
60. Powell I. Prostate cancer among African American men: from the bench to the community. J Natl Med Assoc. 1998;90:S705-9.
61. Roach MI. Is race an independent prognostic factor for survival from prostate cancer? J Natl Med Assoc. 1998;90:S713-9.
62. Fowler J, Terrell F. Survival in blacks and whites after localized treatment for prostate cancer. J Urol. 1996;156:133-6.
63. Morgan T, Jacobson SJ, McCarthy WF, et al. Age-specific reference ranges for prostate specific antigen in black men. N Engl J Med. 1996;335:304-10.
64. Moul J. Use of prostate-specifc antigen in black men: age-adjusted reference ranges for maximal cancer detection. J Natl Med Assoc. 1998;90:S710-2.
65. Eschenbach A, Ho R, Murphy GP, et al. American Cancer Society Guidelines for the Early Detection of Prostate Cancer, 1997 Update. CA Cancer J Clin. 1997;47:261-4.
66. McDonald C. Cancer statistics, 1999: challenges in minority populations. CA Cancer J Clin. 1999;49:6-11.
67. Krieger N. Social class and the black/white crossover in the age-specific incidence of breast cancer: a study linking census-derived data to population-based registry records. Am J Epidemiol. 1990;131:804-14.
68. Erwin D, Spatz T, Tuturro C. Development of an African American role model intervention to increase breast self-examination and mammography. J Cancer Educ. 1992;7:311-9.
69. Schover L. The impact of breast cancer on sexuality, body image, and intimate relationships. CA Cancer J Clin. 1991;41:113-9.
70. Weaver P. Colon cancer in blacks: a disease with worsening prognosis. J Natl Med Assoc. 1991;83:133-6.
71. Royce J, Hymowitz N, Corbett K, et al. Smoking cessation factors among African Americans and whites. Am J Public Health. 1993; 83:220-6.
72. Shervington D. Attitudes and practice of African American women regarding cigarette smoking: implications for intervention. J Natl Med Assoc. 1994;86:337-43.
73. Olsen S, Frank-Stromborg M. Cancer prevention and early detection in ethnically diverse populations. Semin Oncol Nurs. 1993;9:198-209.
74. Kjerulff K, Guzinski GM, Langenberg PW, et al. Hysterectomy and race. Obstet Gynecol. 1993;82:757-64.
75. National Institute of Allergy and Disease. Minorities and HIV infection. Fact Sheet: May 1997.
76. Sullivan P, Chu SY, Fleming PI, Ward JW. Changes in AIDS incidence for men who have sex with men: United States, 1990-1995. AIDS. 1997;11:1641-6.
77. Heckman T, Kelly JA, Bogart LM, et al. Risk differences between African American and white men who have sex with men. J Natl Med Assoc. 1999;91:92-100.
78. Bowser B. African-American culture and AIDS prevention from barrier to ally. West J Med. 1992;157:286-9.
79. Fullilove R, Fullilove MT, Bowsner BP, Gross SA. Risk of sexually transmitted disease among black adolescent crack users in Oakland and San Francisco, California. JAMA. 1990;263:851-5.

80. Centers for Disease Control and Prevention. Primary and secondary syphilis: United States, 1981-1990. MMWR. 1991;40:314-5,332-3.
81. National Drug Control Strategy, 1999. Washington, DC: National Drug Control Office.
82. Brown L. Alcohol abuse prevention in African American communities. J Natl Med Assoc. 1993;85:665-73.
83. Ziedonis D, Rayford BS, Bryant KJ, Rounsaville BJ. Psychiatric co-morbidity in white and African American cocaine addicts seeking substance abuse treatment. Hosp Community Psychiatry. 1994;45:43-8.
84. Boyd C. The antecedents of women's crack cocaine abuse: family substance abuse, sexual abuse, depression and illicit drug use. J Subst Abuse Treat. 1993;10:433-8.
85. Darrow S, Russell M, Cooper ML, Mudar P. Sociodemographic correlates of alcohol consumption among African American and white women. Womens Health. 1992;18:35-51.
86. Rowe D, Grills C. African centered drug treatment: an alternative conceptual paradigm for drug counseling with African-American clients. J Psychoactive Drugs. 1993;25:21-7.
87. Wallace B. Cross-cultural counseling with the chemically dependent: preparing for service delivery within a culture of violence. J Psychoactive Drugs. 1993;25:9-31.
88. Thomas S, Quinn S. The Tuskegee Syphilis Study, 1932 to 1972: implications for HIV education and AIDS risk education programs in the black community. Am J Public Health. 1991;81:1498-1504.

3

Care of Latinos

SUSANA MORALES, MD

In 1999 the Latino population in the United States was estimated at 31.7 million, or 11.7% of the total population. By far, the largest Latino subgroup (65.2%) consists of Mexican Americans or Chicanos, who reside mainly in the Southwest and West. Central and South Americans account for 14.3% of the Latino population; Puerto Ricans comprise 9.6 %; Cuban Americans, who reside mainly in the Southeast, account for 4.3%; and "other Hispanics" make up the remaining 6.6% (1).

Latinos may be of any race. Mexican Americans and Central and South Americans are the most likely to be, at least in part, of American Indian heritage. Due to the importation of slaves, African heritage is common in Latin America (although somewhat less so in Mexico) and in the Caribbean. Significant migrations of Europeans also occurred throughout Latin America, including of course Spaniards and Portuguese but also Germans, Italians, and others. From the Far East, Chinese laborers settled in many regions of the Caribbean, and sizable Japanese communities exist in several Latin American countries.

Immigration of Latinos to the United States has come, notably, in several waves. Large numbers of Mexicans entered the country in the 1970s, and the 1990s saw the immigration of many Central and South Americans. In 2000, three-fifths, or 61%, of Latinos living in the United States were American born (2).

Historical Context

The relations between Latin American countries and the United States have at times been cordial, at others contentious. Besides direct military intervention, the United States has instigated or backed coups and revolutions in several countries.

Mexico

The entire Southwest portion of the United States was once part of Mexico. In 1835, the Mexican province of Texas revolted and was granted its independence a year later. The Republic of Texas continued to engage in border fights with Mexico and soon requested admission to the United States. The annexation of Texas was approved by Congress in 1845. The Mexican-American War (1846-1848), fought over the contested Texas-Mexican border, resulted in the United States acquiring the northern half of Mexico in return for $15 million. Since then, relations between the two countries have been generally good despite some tensions.

United States immigration policy, such as the *bracero* program in the 1960s, has periodically encouraged migration of Mexican workers to their northern neighbor. Recently, however, the number of Mexicans illegally in the United States has raised concern in some quarters.

Puerto Rico

Puerto Rico became a territory of the United States after the Spanish-American War in 1898. Two decades later, in 1917, American citizenship was bestowed on the population by the Jones Act, though a series of military and civilian governors appointed by the mainland continued to head the Puerto Rican government. Not until 1947 were Puerto Ricans given the right to vote for governor. Three years later, however, Puerto Rico was granted Commonwealth status, allowing for limited self-government.

Supporters of an independent Puerto Rico have been active throughout its history, sometimes precipitating violent movements. Several referendums have been held over the years on the subject of Puerto Rico's political status, the most recent in favor of retaining the current Commonwealth form.

The first large-scale migration of Puerto Ricans to the mainland was promoted by the American government in the 1930s. Migration to and from Puerto Rico is facilitated by the fact that all Puerto Ricans are American citizens. The desire to relocate in the United States can be understood when it is realized that the per capita income of Puerto Rico is lower than that of Mississippi, the poorest of the fifty states. Unfortunately, the Puerto Rican population in the United States, concentrated in the urban Northeast, remains characterized by high rates of poverty. Many Americans lack understanding of Puerto Rico's political status, which may be the cause of inaccurate assumptions about, and bias towards, Puerto Ricans seeking health care in mainland institutions (Case 3-1).

Cuba

Spain claimed Cuba in 1492. It soon became a major sugar producer, initially depending heavily on African slaves, then on laborers imported from Mexico and China. The United States tried to purchase Cuba many times during the 1860s, and United States businesses invested heavily in the Cuban economy throughout the later 1800s.

The United States embarked on the Spanish-American War in 1898 for several reasons, among them encouragement by the "yellow press" and the desire for new territory in an age of colonialism. The sinking of the *U.S.S.*

CASE 3-1   A 69-YEAR-OLD PUERTO RICAN MAN SEEKING EMERGENCY CARE

Jose Santiago is a 69-year-old retired municipal worker who, accompanied by his son, presents to a Boston hospital emergency room with a chief complaint of "kidney problems". He had arrived from Puerto Rico earlier that day. He explains that a physician in Puerto Rico had informed him last week that he had kidney failure and needed surgery. Because he also has diabetes and coronary artery disease, he decided to come to Boston, where his son lives, to seek another opinion and then to have the surgery if necessary.

Tests confirm that the patient has an obstructive uropathy due to kidney stones. His creatinine is 6.8; his potassium is 6.0. Mr Santiago and his son agree to the former's admission for further evaluation and management of his hyperkalemia. The emergency room physician comments to the admitting physician, within earshot of the patient's son, "I don't understand how people can come here from Puerto Rico and think they can get treatment when Americans can't even get care." The son confronts the emergency room physician about his insensitivity and lack of knowledge about the status of Puerto Ricans. He leaves with his father to go to another hospital.

Maine, the cause of which is still debated, was another important factor leading to hostilities with Spain.

After the Treaty of Paris ended the War, the United States acquired Cuba and occupied it until 1901. A rebellion, another United States occupation, and a short-lived republican government were followed by a series of rulers, then by an American-sponsored coup by Fulgencio Batista in 1933. Batista oversaw a brutal dictatorship. Poverty and unemployment were severe. Batista's regime ended in a revolution in 1959 led by Fidel Castro. Cuba became a socialist state that nationalized major industry and relied heavily on aid from the Soviet Union. The United States established a Cuban trade embargo in the 1960s and sponsored the unsuccessful attempt by Cuban exiles to invade the Bay of Pigs in 1961 and various attempts to assassinate Castro. Forty years later, relations with Cuba remain strained.

There have been several influxes of Cuban migration to the United States. The first took place during the fall of Batista and the takeover of Castro; many left for economic reasons and settled in South Florida. The second wave of emigrants left Cuba throughout the 1960s for mostly political reasons. Most recently, in the 1970s (the *Mariel* boatlift), many poor and economically disadvantaged persons sought refuge in the United States (3).

Dominican Republic

The island of Hispaniola has had a stormy history. France, Spain, and the United States had either direct or indirect control of the island for much of its history. The Dominican Republic (on the eastern half of the island; the western half is Haiti) was first ruled by Spain, then by a series of dictatorships throughout the 19th century, and was occupied by the United States from 1905 to 1924. An American-backed coup by Rafael Trujillo in 1930 led to a brutal military dictatorship until his assassination in 1961. A democratic election led to the ascent of President Juan Bosch, a democratic socialist. An American-sponsored invasion in 1965-1966 overthrew him. Elections in 1966 installed Joaquin Balaguer as president, a former Trujillo ally and conservative, who ruled until the late 1990s (4).

Dominican immigrants to the United States settle predominantly in the Northeast. Theirs is the fastest growing immigrant community in New York City. Immigration rates have historically fluctuated with poor economic conditions in the Dominican Republic.

Central and South America

Central and South America have also had histories colored by America's "Manifest Destiny" doctrine and military interventions. For example, in the 1970s the Central Intelligence Agency backed a military coup against democratically elected President Salvador Allende of Chile, a democratic socialist. General Augusto Pinochet took control of the government and a military dictatorship subsequently ruled for nearly 20 years. Anastasio Somoza, with United States backing, controlled Nicaragua with an iron hand for decades until the Sandinista revolution. American-backed "contras" fought the Sandinistas for many years until a truce was agreed upon and a democratically elected government was installed. El Salvador, Guatemala, and Honduras have also had long histories of repressive military regimes backed by the United States.

Central and South American immigrants came to the United States mainly in the 1980s, often to escape violence, civil war, and extreme poverty. Many have not been granted legal refugee status and are often ineligible for social services. Central and South Americans have primarily settled in the Northeast and California. These immigrants may have been victims of political repression and torture or have witnessed the torture or execution of family members and friends. Sensitivity and awareness of these traumatic experiences is crucial to compassionate care of these persons.

Demographics and Social Structure

Because the Census Bureau has not adequately collected data on Latino and other minority communities, there has been increased support for representative statistical sampling rather than "head counts". Major national data sets often lack racial and ethnic identifiers, omit major Latino population centers, and usually lack information on Latino/Hispanic subgroups (5). Thus the data below are necessarily incomplete and subject to modification.

The Latino population is younger than the non-Latino white population. Among Latinos, Cubans tend to be older, Mexicans, Puerto Ricans, and other Hispanics younger (5). Latinos are predominantly poor and working class, and are heavily represented in the service and manufacturing industries. The Latino adult labor force participation is the same as for non-Latino whites (67.0% vs. 67.1%). However, Latino men are more likely than non-Latino white men to participate in the labor force (78.4% vs. 74.3%) and Latino women are less likely to work outside the home than non-Latino white women (55.8% vs. 60.3%). Latinos are more likely to be unemployed than non-Latino whites (6.7% vs. 3.6%). Latinos are three times more likely to live in poverty then non-Latino whites (34.4% vs. 10.6%). The poverty rate of Latino families varies by country of origin or descent: Mexican-Americans, 24.4%; Puerto Ricans, 26.7%; Cuban Americans, 11%; Central/South Americans and other Hispanics, 18%. Latino families residing in the United States provide significant financial support for their families abroad.

The Latino community in the United States is educationally disadvantaged. Latinos are more likely than non-Latino whites to never have reached the ninth grade (27.8% vs. 4.5%) (5). Latinos are much less likely than non-Latino whites to have a bachelor's degree or higher (10.9% vs. 27.7%) (1). Latino adults in 1992 had the lowest literacy level of any ethnic group (6). Mexicans had the lowest levels of educational attainment followed by Puerto Ricans, other Latinos, and Cubans (5).

Latinos are highly represented among migrant farm workers, legal seasonal workers who migrate to rural agricultural settings. The migrant worker and his or her family may experience significant stress due to constant dislocations. Health care and education may be fragmented. A network of community-based migrant farm worker clinics is funded by the Health Resource and Services Administration of the Department of Health and Human Services to provide access to health care for this community.

The Latino population of the United States is highly mobile. Travel across the United States-Mexico border is common in both directions, and travel between the United States and more distant or island homelands is a phenomenon sometimes called the "air bridge". This phenomenon differs from immigration earlier in American history, where due to distance, political or religious oppression, or other factors immigrants were less likely to visit or return to their homelands. Latino individuals and families are more likely to travel back and forth to their homelands, particularly during holidays, summertime, and at times of bereavement, illness, or family crisis. These visits may serve to buttress extended family ties and provide a relief from social isolation, economic deprivation, and racism experienced in the United States.

Some Latinos travel to their homelands for medical treatment they have been unable to obtain in the United States. Some pursue health care in the United States, often perceived to be of superior quality to that available abroad, but desire death or burial in their nation of origin. Persons residing in border regions may use medications obtained in foreign countries, often available without prescription. (Of note, some medications available in Latin America have been reported to come from outdated pharmaceutical stocks.) Travel to the homeland may lead to interruptions of schooling or medical treatment. Experiences of health care in the homeland may influence or affect expectations of the health care system in the United States.

Immigration Policy and Impact on Health Care

United States immigration policy has had a powerful impact on Latino health and access to health care. Latinos are more likely to be foreign born than the non-Latino white population. There are an estimated 3.5 million Latinos who do not have legal status in the United States. Immigrants granted legal residence since 1996 cannot receive Medicaid for 5 years. Accepting entitlement benefits for themselves or their children may jeopardize the opportunity to gain permanent legal status due to Immigration and Naturalization Service (INS) rules that until recently designated recipients of entitlements a "public charge" (7). Enrollment of legal resident or American citizen children in the federally funded Child Health Insurance Program (CHIP) has been very low in many Latino communities. Statutes and laws such as Proposition 187 in California, which mandated reporting of even suspected undocumented persons by employees of any publicly funded agency or institution, including schools, hospitals and clinics, have led to fear of INS involvement when seeking health care services.

Acculturation

The encounter with a new culture may affect several aspects of psychological function, including language use, behavior, sense of identity, attitudes, and stress levels. Some people adapt and integrate their previous attitudes and practices into the new culture; others may reject the "new" entirely.

One of the most easily measured changes produced by acculturation is language use. Some Hispanic immigrants completely shift to English; others become bilingual; others keep their native language as primary. Besides language, acculturation has been shown to affect, for example, mental health, levels of social support, alcoholism and drug use, political and social attitudes, and health behaviors such as cigarette smoking and the use of preventive cancer screening practices.

Social Patterns and Family Structure

Latinos are less likely to be married (51.3%) than non-Latino whites (57.6%). Latino households are more likely than white households to be headed by a single female (23.7 vs. 13%) or a single male (22.7% vs. 6.1%). The poverty rate among Latino single female households is 43.7%. Latino families and households are larger than white families (5). Families may be divided by migration; some members may pioneer immigration to the United States and then bring children, spouses, and other family members later. In some urban areas, especially those hard hit by cocaine and HIV, grandparents may have a significant role in childcare, which may place significant financial and emotional stress on them. The process of acculturation (see above), especially its intergenerational characteristics, may place significant stress on family members, particularly concerning issues of sexuality, education, and autonomy.

The extended family often has a significant role in Latino health-related decision-making. Family members may pose many questions to providers about health care issues or the condition of the patient. Issues of patient confidentiality may conflict with the demonstrated concern of families; that is, the focus on the family rather than the individual as a fundamental unit may conflict with traditional American approaches to health care decision-making. Latino families may also have a strong desire to protect the elderly from bad news, a course of action sometimes viewed by the physician as harmful to the patient. This may also conflict with current American biomedical values related to disclosure and informed consent. Physicians should ask patients about what information can and cannot be divulged. Careful alliance with family members and the patient will facilitate the decision-making process.

For several reasons, family members should not be used as interpreters. Patient confidentiality is necessarily breached. Professional interpreters have been trained in the translation of medical terminology. Family members may omit (intentionally or unintentionally) important or difficult information. Case 3-2 gives an example of the pitfalls of using family members as interpreters.

CASE 3-2   A 52-YEAR-OLD DOMINICAN WOMAN WHO PRESENTS WITH HER SISTER AS INTERPRETER

Rita Sanchez is a 52-year-old Dominican woman who has recently joined her sister in the United States. She visits her primary care physician because of recent unexplained weight loss. She has no specific symptoms and claims to be eating adequately. Extensive evaluation, including thyroid function tests, chest radiography, colonoscopy, abdominal CT scan, stool cultures, and mammography, does not reveal any specific causes of weight loss. The patient denies symptoms of depression through her sister, who serves as interpreter.

On Miss Sanchez's follow-up visit, her physician decides to use a trained interpreter to obtain a more detailed medical history. With her sister out of the room, Miss Sanchez now reveals that she is concerned about her spiritual well-being. In the Dominican Republic she had an altar in her home at which she practiced Santeria. Miss Sanchez's sister, however, refuses to allow an altar or any other expression of Santeria in her home. After discussion between the physician and sister, the patient is allowed to renew her practice of Santeria and soon regains her weight.

DISCUSSION

This case illustrates two points. The first is the importance of asking the patient about his or her degree of acculturation. The second demonstrates one of the pitfalls of using family members as interpreters.

Gender Roles and Sexuality

Latino Women

Traditional Latino female roles include devotion to home, family, and children; self-sacrifice in the interests of the family; care of the elderly; and subservience or docility. Some traditional Latino men oppose their wife's employment outside the home and the higher education of female children.

Latino women may thus have decreased financial autonomy. On the other hand, Latino women are often the "unrecognized" managers and decision-makers in the home, and in child rearing. Women are likely to be the prime health care decision-makers in Latino families. Motherhood is highly valued, and children are felt to be especially precious.

Female virginity is often highly valued in unmarried women, and female sexual fidelity is especially valued within marriage. Unmarried Hispanic women in one cohort had fewer sexual partners than Hispanic men, but condom use was involved less frequently (8), possibly because women felt embarrassed or humiliated when purchasing condoms. Issues of shame or embarrassment about sexual matters may also influence Latino women accessing gynecologic care or negotiating condom use. Some women may view examination by male physicians as overly intrusive. Acculturation and intergenerational differences in perspectives on female sexual activity, especially among young women, may be the source of significant stress within Latino families.

Latino Men

Traditional Latino male roles are characterized by the importance of *machismo,* which includes accepting responsibility, having a strong work ethic, providing for one's family; physical strength, and courage or daring. *Machismo* may also include complete decision-making powers and control over family finances and family members and their actions, in particular over female members and their sexual morality and reputations. Male marital infidelity may be tacitly supported by being attributed to *machismo* as a display of virility, although this may contrast with commitment and devotion to family.

One study of condom use among Hispanic men demonstrated that 38% of subjects reported a secondary female sexual partner in the year prior to the interview, and multiple barriers to condom use. Hispanics are reported to have negative attitudes about condoms and are less likely to believe that condoms protect against HIV infection (8). Sexual side effects of medications may be of particular concern to Latinos, and discussion of these side effects may be difficult. Commitment to work and self-sacrifice on behalf of family, and the need to demonstrate physical strength and to tolerate pain or work without complaint, may contribute to delays in seeking health care among Latino men. For example, Latino men are much less likely to have seen a physician within the past year, and almost half did not have a regular doctor; 57% did not get routine preventive care in the last year (9).

Domestic Violence

Issues of power and traditional gender roles may result in complex attitudes toward domestic violence. On the one hand, protection of the family is an important value; on the other, control over decisions and the importance of male power in the family unit may conflict with this value. Jealousy and extreme concern about female sexual virtue may be important components of battering syndromes. A Latino woman who is involved in a violent relationship may experience strong family and cultural pressures to remain in that relationship. The rate of domestic violence for Latino women is comparable to that for non-Latino whites; the rate is highest for black women (8/1000 for whites, 7/1000 for Latinos, 12/1000 for blacks) (10).

Homosexuality

Homosexuality among Latinos has historically been viewed as negative and shameful. Stigma about homosexual behavior may contribute to the higher rates of bisexuality reported among Latino men who have sex with men. Latino men who have sex with men may be especially uncomfortable reporting such behavior to their health care providers. Some Latino men who are the inserting partner in anal intercourse with other men may not identify this as a homosexual practice. Latino men who have sex with both women and men may identify themselves as heterosexual. A careful, specific sexual history is therefore an especially important part of risk assessment and tailored education for Latino males.

Health Beliefs and Practices

Cultural Attitudes

Latinos traditionally value *personalismo,* the trust and rapport that is established with others by developing warm, friendly, and personal relationships. Thus Latino patients often prefer health care providers who take a personal interest in their lives. Patients may embrace their doctors and bring them gifts of food or other tokens of appreciation. *Respeto* (respect) and *dignidad* (dignity) are other valued signs of esteem. For example, professional attire is valued; addressing individuals by their formal names (Mr/Mrs; Senor/Senora), especially for older patients, is a sign of correct behavior (11).

Disease Causation

Latinos may believe that several illnesses stem from *susto* (fright). Some Latinos, particularly those of Mexican heritage, subscribe to a hot-and-cold theory of disease causation and treatment. This theory may derive from the Hippocratic concept of bodily humors in which a proper balance of these humors is vital to health (14); others feel there is evidence of such a belief in Pre-Columbian cultures. This concept is not related to temperature but rather to the intrinsic qualities of certain times of day or foods; for example, ice cream is a hot food and most meats are considered cold (12).

Other beliefs about disease causation include exposure to cold or wet, or allowing air to blow on one's head. Some less serious pains are ascribed to "gases" or "air" in the body. Practitioners of *espiritismo* and Santeria, and some others, may ascribe illness to a spell (*un trabajo*) or the "evil eye" cast by someone who is jealous or envious of the affected person. An old injury may lead to cancer or chronic pain. *Caida de mollera* (fallen fontanelle) may cause illness in children. Abdominal pain may be caused by *empacho* (usually used to describe an upset stomach or "clogging" of the intestines); treatment is sometimes with cathartics, sometimes with mercurials. Nutrition and rest are viewed as important illness prevention measures.

Stress is clearly linked to physical illness in the view of many Latinos. *Ataque de nervios* (attack of nerves) is an example of a culture-bound concept of illness that overlaps with panic attacks and anxiety disorders (12a).

Traditional Healing Practices and Biomedical Treatments

The use of alternative and complementary healing practices among Latinos has been well documented. Most practitioners of nontraditional healing practices use them as an adjunct to biomedical treatments rather than as substitutes. Many homes in Latin America traditionally had at least two gardens: a vegetable and fruit garden, and a curative herb garden. Many Latinos today use traditional methods of healing, some involving patent medicines that are heavily marketed in the Spanish-language media. These medicines are found in local stores devoted to such "natural" remedies or in *botanicas* (shops where religious and spiritual products are available).

Herbs used in Mexican American communities include *yerbabuena* (*Mentha spicata*), *ruda* (*Ruta graveolens*), *albacar* (*Ocimum basilicum*), and *altamisa* (*Tanacetum parthenium*). These agents may have antibacterial and analgesic effects (13). In addition to traditional herbal remedies, frequently ingested in the form of teas, other substances such as mercury may be ingested (14). Special foods, such as soups and juices, may be viewed as having healing properties.

Candles and prayer, cleansing of the home, and ritual baths are believed by some Latinos to aid the healing process. Massages (*sobos*) are often an important part of caring for the sick. Twenty-three percent of Latinos use herbal medicines as opposed to 12% of non-Latino whites; 31% of Latinos use home remedies; and 8% of Latinos use chiropractic services (10). Many Latinos also use the services of traditional healers (*curanderos, espiritistas, santeros*), who, like modern physicians, may specialize in one condition or disease. In some regions, particularly the rural Southwest, women may use traditional lay midwives at childbirth.

Some Latinos have serious concerns about biomedical treatments and what they consider their artificial or unnatural origins. Some people expect injections or intravenous medications rather than pills or capsules, in part due to practices in their nation of origin. During illness, Latinos may work through a hierarchy of help—first traditional home remedies (especially for common complaints like upper respiratory infections), then traditional healers, and finally physicians and other biomedical providers. Many Latino patients use traditional and biomedical treatments simultaneously, though many will not volunteer this information to their providers (Case 3-3).

Fatalism is a potential problem. Some Latinos feel that certain illnesses, such as cancer, are unlikely to be cured, and thus will reject treatment.

Religion and Spirituality

Participation in religious services is an important source of social support. Religious practice may also influence health through psychodynamic pathways. Attendance at religious services has been linked to a protective effect on mortality in the elderly (15).

Faith has traditionally played a large role in Latino cultural and community life. Clergy and other spiritual leaders are often important sources of advice and counsel. Prayer is viewed by many as an important adjunct to medical care. Most Latinos are Roman Catholic, but an increasing number

---

**CASE 3-3   A 47-YEAR-OLD CUBAN WOMAN WHO USES
TRADITIONAL TREATMENT**

---

*Maria Clemente is a 47-year-old Cuban who has severe post-
herpetic neuralgia. She is treated with gabapentin and narcotics
but is concerned about their side effects. A return visit reveals a
fine blue pattern on her skin over the area where she had the
herpes zoster. On closer inspection the blue pattern proves to be
ink from a prayer written over the dermatome by a traditional
healer.*

*Her physician acknowledges the intervention and expresses the
hope that it will help the pain. She also informs Miss Clemente
that this traditional treatment can be used along with the prescribed medications. Miss Clemente has felt better since the
prayer inscription, and this allows the physician to decrease her
dose of narcotics and results in fewer side effects.*

DISCUSSION

This case illustrates the importance of acknowledging the
patient's use of complementary therapies. The physician's
acknowledgement allowed the patient to benefit from both
traditional treatment and prescribed medication.

---

are Protestants (e.g., Latino Methodists, particularly in Texas). Some have
joined evangelical Protestant sects. A substantial number of Jews settled in
parts of Latin America (e.g., Cuba) and have since immigrated to the
United States.

Religious proscriptions may contribute to the lower rates of suicide among
Latinos. Faith and religious awakening or conversion may be critical to some
individuals being able to recover from a family or health crisis or addiction.
A *promesa* is the promise to God or to a saint of devotion and sacrifice in
return for the gift of recovery from illness. A person fulfilling a *promesa* may
dress entirely in white for a year or longer. Many Latinos wear crucifixes or
scapulars as symbols of faith and sometimes as a protection against evil or
illness. Arranging for Last Rites or the Sacrament of the Sick may be important to a hospitalized ill or dying patient of Catholic background.

Interestingly, anticlericalism has been a historical political trend in much of Latin America, a result of the Catholic Church's perceived alliance with ruling oligarchies. Liberation theology is a movement of some church members in impoverished areas of Latin America that has promoted the role of religion in social change movements and empowerment of the poor; for example, some activists in liberation theology became leaders in the Sandinista revolution in Nicaragua.

Some Latino subgroups (particularly those from the Caribbean) practice Santeria, an Afro-Caribbean religion synthesizing African religion and Christianity, or *espritismo* (spiritualism). These religious belief systems also include healing practices. Santeria was illegal in most of Latin America, and a tradition of secrecy has persisted; patients or family members are not likely to confide its practice to health care providers (see Case 3-2). Some devotees of Santeria may wear characteristic beads of colors associated with their patron saint or African religious figures.

Diet

The traditional Latino diet exerts a protective effect on Latino health, probably contributing to the Latino health "paradox" (described later in this chapter). For example, compared with blacks and non-Latino whites, Latinos have the lowest fat intakes (16). The dietary habits of Latino subgroups vary. For example, Mexican Americans ingest more corn, beans, chili peppers, and tomatoes; Puerto Ricans and Cubans eat more rice, beans, and *viandas* (starchy root vegetables); Cubans eat more fruits; Puerto Ricans drink more milk; all subgroups enjoy cheese. Mexican American adults eat more protein-rich foods than Cubans and Puerto Ricans. Few Latinos eat fruits or vegetables more than once a day. Lard is used often by all groups for cooking (17). Mexican Americans tend to have lower cholesterol but higher total fat, saturated fat, and monounsaturated fat intake than Puerto Ricans and older Cuban Americans (18). The nutritional advantage appears to wane with acculturation. First-generation Mexican American women have a markedly better diet than that of the second-generation, whose diet more closely approximates that of white women (19).

Latinos are at higher risk for hunger. The Third National Health and Nutrition Examination Survey (NHANES III), a cross-sectional representative survey sample of the civilian noninstitutionalized population, defined "food insufficiency" as "the respondent reported that the family 'sometimes' or 'often' did not get enough food to eat". Latinos may be less likely to apply for food stamps because of fear and distrust of interaction with the government. Traditional attitudes about self-sufficiency and the humiliation of dependence may also discourage accessing services.

Communication and Language

Spanish and English

Most Latinos speak Spanish at home. Rates of limited English proficiency are highest in first-generation immigrants, even those who have been in the United States for many years. Barriers to English language acquisition include low literacy and educational levels (in any language), poor access to English-language instruction, and immersion in work and home with little time for additional study. Second-generation Latinos are likely to be bilingual, although some begin to lose Spanish-language facility and may have a limited vocabulary and knowledge of grammar. For many, English-language acquisition is linked to citizenship application. Insistence on English facility and the detailed questioning on American history may be barriers to citizenship even to long-term residents of the United States.

Some persons of Latin American origin may not speak Spanish, or may speak it with decreased proficiency, due to their indigenous origins. Persons of Native American origin who speak an indigenous language as their primary tongue populate much of Mexico and Central and South America.

Nonverbal Communication

Nonverbal as well as verbal expressions of personal warmth and caring (smiles, handshakes, and sometimes hugs) on the part of health care providers are important priorities for most Latino patients. On the other hand, *respeto* (respectfulness) is also valued, and overly familiar or patronizing behavior may be experienced negatively. Among some Latinos, eye contact may not occur, or may occur less often, especially among persons of low socioeconomic status or educational level, or if the patient disagrees with or does not understand the doctor's plan of treatment.

Health Issues

Overall Health Status

Heart disease and cancer are the two leading causes of death among all Americans. In 1996, the leading causes of death for Latino women were cerebrovascular disease, diabetes, and accidents and unintentional injuries; for Latino men, accidents and unintentional injuries, HIV infection, and homicide. The Latino age-adjusted death rate is lower than that for whites (366/100,000 vs. 277/100,000), but Latinos and blacks are more likely than whites to report fair or poor health status (10).

The National Health Interview Study analyzed Latino subgroup data from 1992 to 1995. Puerto Ricans were much more likely to have an activity limitation (20%) than Mexicans and Cubans (15%), to report being in fair or poor health, to have seen a doctor in the past year, to have days spent in bed due to illness, and to have had a hospital stay. Puerto Ricans were more likely to smoke than members of other Latino subgroups (20). Latinos and blacks with chronic diseases such as hypertension, diabetes, heart disease, and arthritis reported worse functional status than whites, although this was closely tied to socioeconomic status (21).

The Latino Paradox

Many studies have linked low socioeconomic status (SES) to poor health outcomes. Yet Latino populations have very low SES and *lower* mortality rates for cancer and cardiovascular disease and *lower* infant mortality rates. This has been called the *Latino paradox.* The Latino paradox does not apply equally to all Latino subgroups: Puerto Ricans, for example, have higher infant mortality and maternal mortality rates (comparable to those for blacks), as well as more negative health indicators, than other Latino subgroups such as Mexican Americans.

Possible explanations for the Latino paradox include positive health behaviors and risks (lower smoking and alcohol consumption) and protective "genetic factors". Other researchers, however, theorize that the paradox is rather the combination of two factors: 1) immigrants moving to the United States tend to be younger and healthier, and 2) back-migration. Back-migration, also called the *salmon hypothesis,* suggests that Latinos return to their homeland when they are older and therefore are not counted in mortality statistics in the United States. Abraido-Lanza and co-workers tested this theory by linking large population based data sets. Their findings did not support back-migration as lower mortality rates persisted among Puerto Ricans and Cubans (Puerto Rican death rates are included in the vital statistics for Americans, and Cuban Americans are usually unable to return to their homelands) and among American-born Latinos (22).

Other characteristics that may account for lower mortality rates for Latinos include increased family support and extensive social networks (22). The protective effect appears to wane with length of time in the United States; for example, Mexican immigrants have lower infant mortality rates than American-born Mexicans. The process of acculturation generally includes increased rates of tobacco, alcohol, and illicit drug use. More-acculturated Latinos are likely to have had longer exposure to environmental toxins, to have been more frequently subjected to discrimination, and to have disrupted social relationships and networks (20).

Reproductive Health, Contraception, and Abortion

Data from 1995 show that Latino teenagers are more likely to be sexually active, to become pregnant, and to carry the pregnancy to term than non-Latino white teenagers. Lifetime pregnancy rates for Latin women are higher. Induced abortion rates are lower (23).

Disease Prevention

Latino elderly are much less likely to receive immunizations for pneumococcal pneumonia or influenza than non-Latino whites. Latinos have decreased access to cancer screening such as mammography, Pap smears, and fecal occult blood testing or sigmoidoscopy (24). Low rates of Pap smears may reflect culturally based beliefs about cervical cancer causation related to morality and sexual behavior (25).

Violence

Minority adults are more likely to have been victims of violent crime than non-Latino whites (Latinos, 43%; blacks, 49%; whites, 38%). Minority adults are more than two times more likely to say they have been affected by violence than whites, that they fear crime, have been victimized, or know someone who has been assaulted. Young minorities have high rates of death from homicide and legal intervention. In 1996, the death rate from homicide per 100,000 was 123 for blacks, 49 for Latinos, and 14 for whites.

Work-Related Injuries and Automobile Accidents

Minorities are over-represented in hazardous industries and occupations. Latino and other minority workers have been shown to have higher rates of fatal occupational injuries and may be at high risk for occupational disease, although data are scarce in this area (26). Latinos were over-represented among workers in high-risk industries in California who were found to have lead poisoning (27).

Latino populations have higher death rates from automobile accidents than whites or blacks. Studies link this higher accident and death rate to alcohol-related injuries, particularly among adolescents and young adults (significantly higher rates of drunk driving), and low levels of community education, awareness, and use of safety belts and child car seats. The influence of gender roles (e.g., the use of seat belts being viewed as a nonmasculine behavior) has also been reported (28).

Specific Diseases

Obesity

The Behavioral Risk Factor Surveillance System (BRFSS) reported increasing rates of obesity, particularly among Hispanics (29). Latinos have higher rates of obesity than non-Latino whites. Minority women in the BRFSS were the most likely to be inactive, though the US Women's Determinants Study showed that Latin women were more active than other groups in some types of physical activity (30). Cultural norms about body image and exercise may influence levels of obesity.

Diabetes

Latinos are estimated to have two to four times the prevalence of diabetes mellitus of non-Latino whites. The San Antonio Heart Study showed that younger Latinos were likely to have decreased sensitivity to insulin, higher insulin levels, and higher rates of NIDDM (31). One large population based study showed that Latinos were much more likely to have markedly elevated fasting plasma glucose levels than non-Latino whites; these levels were exceeded only by American Indians (32).

Data from the Hispanic Established Populations for Epidemiologic Studies of the Elderly showed a prevalence of diabetes mellitus of 22% among Mexican American elderly, with high rates of obesity, diabetes-related complications, and use of diabetic medications. Rates of myocardial infarction, cerebrovascular accident, hypertension, angina, cancer, depression, disability, incontinence, visual impairment, and hospitalization were higher in diabetics (33). The incidence of type 2 diabetes in Mexican Americans in the San Antonio Heart Study is rising rapidly (34).

Hypertension

Latinos have lower or equal rates of hypertension compared with non-Latino whites. However, of hypertensive subjects studied in the Hispanic HANES, less than 10% of Latino men had controlled blood pressure (35).

Cardiovascular Disease

Latinos have cardiovascular death rates comparably lower than non-Hispanic whites (36). Mexican-born immigrants, despite poverty and low educational levels, have lower cardiovascular death rates than American-born Mexicans and non-Latino whites, possibly because of differences in diet (rich in fruits and vegetables, low in fat), smoking rates in women (lower), and level of physical activity (higher). Racial and ethnic disparities in the use of cardiovascular procedures have been documented for minorities across most insurance classes, although not always in private insurance (37). Latino women with myocardial infarctions have significantly lower death rates than non-Latino women (38).

Cancer

Overall rates of cancer among Latinos are lower than among non-Latino whites. Latinos have increased rates of invasive cervical cancer; Latinos have lower colorectal cancer survival rates than non-Latino whites. Hispanic women are more likely to be diagnosed in late stages of breast cancer compared with non-Hispanic white women. Physicians recommend mammography less often with Latin women than with non-Latino patients. Hispanic cancer patients have higher out-of-pocket expenses (see Financial Barriers below) and report more difficulty getting to chemotherapy or radiation treatment centers due to travel problems (e.g., no access to an automobile) (39). Hispanic cancer patients, in particular, had less pain relief and less adequate analgesia in the Eastern Cooperative Group Minority Outpatient Pain Study (40).

HIV/AIDS and Other Sexually Transmitted Diseases

Nineteen percent of the 415,864 cases of AIDS diagnosed from 1991 to 1996 were in Latinos, of whom 67% were American-born or resided in Puerto Rico. Latino women are particularly hard hit. Puerto Rican born men with AIDS are more likely to have been infected through injection drug use; men of Cuban, Mexican, or Central or South American birth were more likely to be infected by men who have sex with other men. A trend of increasing AIDS cases among foreign-born Latino men and women (mostly from heterosexual transmission) and among American-born Latinos (mostly in injection drug users and men who have sex with men) has been observed. Most foreign-born Latinos probably became infected in the United States. Foreign-born Latino women and those of "low acculturation" may be less likely to use condoms and thus be at increased risk for HIV infection.

Injection drug use is more common among Puerto Ricans than other Latino subgroups and this may be linked to higher HIV rates in this subgroup (41). Latinos and blacks have higher death rates from HIV than non-Latino white persons. In 1995, the principal cause of death among young Latinos was HIV disease, with comparatively high rates of heterosexual transmission and higher rates in men who have sex with men than among non-Latino whites. Minority patients have been in the past less likely to receive antiretroviral therapy (42).

Despite strong evidence of decreased perinatal transmission of HIV with the use of antiretroviral therapy, minority women, including Latino women, are much less likely to adhere to antiretrovirals during pregnancy (43). Women at high risk for HIV infection include those under severe social stress (e.g., homelessness, drug addiction). Active coping styles, higher self-esteem, and less-frequent drug use decrease risk among this group.

Many women are at risk for HIV due to the sexual or drug use activities of their male partners. Traditional gender roles, low levels of power in couple relationships, socioeconomic reliance on the male partner, male objections to the use of condoms, and severe life and socioeconomic stresses and chaotic living situations decrease condom use. Many women also have misconceptions about the use and efficacy of condoms (44). An HIV program consisting of risk reduction workshops and community prevention events decreased unprotected intercourse and other risk factors in a high-risk inner city population (45).

Although other sexually transmitted diseases do not appear to have a higher incidence in Latinos, hepatitis C is more common in Latinos than in blacks or non-Latino whites (46).

Mental Health and Substance Use

Moderate-to-severe depressive symptoms and stress are more prevalent among Latinos than among non-Latino whites; 34% of Latinos had such stress compared with 26% of non-Latino whites (10). However, a study of very low income Hispanic migrant farm workers showed lower rates of lifetime psychiatric disorders compared with Mexican Americans and the United States population as a whole. Social support and strong family ties and group identity most likely account for these lower rates (47). In an insured national cohort, black and Latino patients were less likely to use mental health services (48). Bilingual mental health services are in high demand but frequently unavailable.

Overall, minorities are less likely to use illicit drugs than non-Latino whites (31% of blacks, 26% of Hispanics, 38% of whites). Lifetime exposure to tobacco is highest among non-Latino whites. Smoking rates are similar across all groups; Latino women, however, are the least likely to have smoked within the past year. A lower percentage of Latinos and blacks use alcohol compared with non-Latino whites, but minorities have higher alcohol-related death rates and illnesses (10).

Asthma

Homa et al (49) analyzed vital statistics data from 1990-1995 and found that asthma-related mortality in the United States is highest among Puerto Ricans and African Americans (Table 3-1). Rates of death of Puerto Ricans were highest in the Northeast (47.8/million). These data further support the heterogeneity of Latino groups and analysis of data by Latino subgroups. The prevalence of asthma and asthma mortality are higher among Caribbean-born Latinos, in particular Puerto Ricans, when compared with other Latino subgroups, even in different subgroups sharing the same environment (50).

Table 3-1 Age-Adjusted Annual Asthma-Related Mortality Rates for Three Latino Subgroups, Non-Latino Whites, and Non-Latino Blacks in the United States, 1990-1995

Demographic Group	Annual Asthma-Related Mortality Rate (Per Million)
Puerto Ricans	40.9
Cuban Americans	15.8
Mexican Americans	9.2
Non-Latino whites	14.7
Non-Latino blacks	38.1

Data from Homa DM, Mannino DM, Lara M. Asthma mortality in U.S. Hispanics of Mexican, Puerto Rican, and Cuban heritage, 1990-1995. Am J Respir Crit Care Med. 2000;161:504-9.

Latino children have been reported to have difficulty accessing care for asthma and obtaining preventive medical treatment, and are less likely to receive nebulizer equipment upon hospital discharge. A group of Los Angeles based pediatricians reported marked problems with health care access, poor patient and family understanding of prevention and treatment strategies, poorly coordinated health services, and nonadherence to care (51).

Barriers to Access to Health Care

Financial Barriers

Financial and nonfinancial barriers limit access to health care. Lack of access to health care is clearly linked to socioeconomic status. The high rate of poverty in the Latino population contributes markedly to decreased access to care, but even employed non-poor Latinos have high rates of uninsuredness. Latinos are the ethnic group most likely to be uninsured and underinsured. They are over-represented in service and laborer sectors, which often do not provide coverage to their employees. Some states prevent working poor adults, even those with extremely low incomes, from obtaining Medicaid in spite of federal policy that could allow such an option. Approximately 30% of uninsured Latinos live in Florida or Texas, both of which have limited Medicaid programs. Many Latinos are American citizens or legal permanent residents and thus are eligible for federal entitlement programs but are not receiving them. Private purchase of health insurance policies is prohibitively expensive for poor and many Latino families (7).

Latino immigrants are very likely to lack health insurance, particularly recent immigrants. In addition, there are an estimated 3.5 million noncitizens who do not have legal status in the United States and cannot legally access benefits. Undocumented persons disproportionately utilize safety net institutions for their care. Fear of the Immigration and Naturalization Service may make even eligible immigrants turn away from Medicaid or CHIP (7).

Language Barriers

Latinos report major problems in communicating with their doctors and other health care providers. Data from the 1990 census revealed that almost half of Latino respondents spoke English less than very well and 25% spoke English not well or not at all (52). Given the tremendous growth in the Hispanic community over the past decade and the high percentage of recent immigrants, as well as known census undercounts of Latinos and other immigrant groups, it is likely that the percentage of Latinos who do not speak English well is even higher than reported. Even Latinos who report fair English ability are more likely than other ethnic groups to have difficulty communicating with and understanding physicians. A third of Latinos, as opposed to 16% of whites, reported communication problems with doctors. Latinos who mainly speak Spanish at home are the most likely to report difficulties (43%) (53).

Latinos with limited English proficiency reported fewer doctor visits than native English-speaking patients, although an analysis of the National Medical Expenditure Survey of 1987 did not show a difference between these groups. Emergency department patients whose first language was not English had lower patient satisfaction (54). In one study, patients with language barriers were less likely to receive a follow-up appointment following emergency room visits (55). Waxman and Levitt reported that increased numbers of diagnostic tests for the evaluation of abdominal pain were ordered in the emergency department for non-English speaking patients (56), and Hampers and collaborators also documented that a physician-family language barrier was associated with a higher rate of diagnostic testing and increased numbers of emergency room visits (57).

Some data point to improved health outcomes when there is language concordance between physician and patient. Unfortunately, interpreter services are unavailable in many clinical settings, and Latino physicians and other providers are under-represented in health care fields. Latino patients who did not have an interpreter when they thought one was important were less satisfied with the doctor-patient encounter. Latino patients sometimes do not ask for interpreters because of respect for the doctor.

Inadequate access to professional interpreters, and the resulting use of family members, friends, even persons in the waiting room, as interpreters, all of whom have no medical interpretation training, contribute to communication problems in the physician-patient relationship. Physicians and other health care providers with some knowledge of Spanish but incomplete bilingualism may attempt communication without the use of interpreters. Though the effort may be appreciated by the patient, miscommunication is not uncommon and potentially dangerous. For example, some Latinos refer to *fatiga,* which sometimes means "shortness of breath" or "asthma", whereas providers may assume the word to mean "fatigue" or "tiredness"; and *nervios* (literally, "nervousness") can refer to a slight anxiety or to paranoid schizophrenia.

The persistence of language barriers to access to quality health care can be traced to multiple causes, including inadequate or no reimbursement for providing bilingual services; institutional lack of commitment; nonexistence of structures to facilitate interpreter services; provider indifference, sense of helplessness, or burnout; patient and community lack of awareness or empowerment to demand such services, English-only legislation, and political biases.

Discrimination

Racism and discrimination can influence access to care, timeliness of care, and quality of care. Latino and other minority patients are more likely to believe they would have received better care if they were of another race. Latino patients may perceive English-only signage and written materials and a lack of Spanish-speaking personnel as unwelcoming or discriminatory (10). Disparities in clinical outcomes and process of care have been well documented; for example, Latinos with long bone fractures were two times more likely than whites to receive *no* pain medication in a California emergency room (58).

Low Educational and Literacy Levels

Low educational levels and low literacy contribute to difficulties in keeping track of appointments, understanding medication instructions, and understanding information about health conditions.

Logistic Barriers

Transportation is a significant barrier to accessing care, especially for individuals with chronic illness. Latino cancer patients reported difficulty finding someone to drive them to chemotherapy treatments (39). Rural Latinos may have to travel long distances for health care. Even in urban areas, location of health services outside public transportation areas may present severe barriers to access. Regions with less-developed public transportation systems (e.g., California) provide special hardships for poor Latinos who cannot afford automobiles.

Many individuals, particularly women, report delaying care due to responsibilities for children and for the care of sick or elderly family members. Bringing children to visits may be an additional expense but the only option for some women. Paying babysitters may be a severe hardship and not a real option.

Many physician offices are only open during usual business hours, so that working people may not be able to access them easily. Because, as mentioned earlier, a disproportionate number of Latinos work in the service and labor sectors, days lost from work are generally unpaid. More frequent use of the emergency room by Latinos may be linked to its more convenient hours (around the clock) as well as to the lack of health insurance.

Enhancing Compliance

Barriers to adherence to medically prescribed treatment include cost of medication(s), poor communication between patient and physician, illiteracy (e.g., patient cannot read pill bottle), and health beliefs (e.g., patient is afraid of too many medications or operations). Establishing a trusting physician-patient relationship where diagnoses and treatments are explained as concisely as possible can overcome patient fears, but patients may still conceal disagreements about diagnoses, evaluation, or treatment out of respect for the provider. Therefore physicians should repeatedly ask patients if they understand what they have been told and invite them to express opinions or feelings about their diagnosis, care, and treatment. Patient confidentiality must be respected, but engaging family members in an alliance may be helpful. Questions such as "May I speak to your daughter about your health and condition?" is often taken as a sign of caring.

Community resources may be available to provide adjunct services in a culturally competent fashion. For example, the Visiting Nurse Service of New York has programs for Spanish-, Chinese-, and Russian-speaking patients, with bilingual nurses and patient education materials. Prescriptions for Spanish-speaking patients should always have "Label in Spanish" written on them, because many pharmacies, particularly those in Latino neighborhoods, have computer programs that translate the prescription information. The Latino media, particularly print and radio, often provide significant amounts of health information, signaling the community's interest in this area.

Physicians may also find assistance in dealing with difficult clinical issues from community-based agencies that specialize in serving Latinos. Housing, social services, educational, cultural, faith-based, and other organizations may provide consultations for understanding health dilemmas from a culturally specific aspect. These organizations can often provide the physician with an explanation or understanding of Latino traditions or behaviors or beliefs that will aid him in providing proper patient care.

Summary of High-Risk Conditions and Other Health Issues in Latinos

Be on the alert for presenting signs of the following conditions. Keep in mind that history-taking must take into account cultural differences that may otherwise mislead the physician (e.g., reluctance to talk about sexual activity).

➤ Nutritional problems
  • Latinos at higher risk for hunger ("food insufficiency")

➤ Injuries
  • Accidents and unintentional injuries
  • Occupational injuries

(Cont'd.)

Summary of High-Risk Conditions and Other Health Issues in Latinos (continued)

➤ Diabetes
- 2 to 4 times more prevalent than among non-Latino whites
- Decreased sensitivity to insulin
- Higher insulin levels
- Higher rates of NIDDM

➤ Obesity

➤ Cancer
- Overall rates of cancer are lower among Latinos than among non-Latino whites
- However, special concerns regarding survival rates and cancer stage at presentation are as follows:
- *Breast cancer*—Latino women tend to present with more advanced stages of breast cancer than non-Latino white women
- *Cervical cancer*—Latino women have higher rates of cervical cancer than non-Latino white women
- *Colorectal cancer*—Latinos have lower survival rates

➤ HIV/AIDS
- Leading cause of death among young Latinos
- Latinos comprise 19% of total AIDS cases while representing 12% of total U.S. population
- Latinos are less likely to use antiretroviral therapy during pregnancy

➤ Depression
- Moderate-to-severe depression is more prevalent among Latinos than among non-Latino whites

➤ Asthma
- More prevalent among Puerto Ricans than among non-Latino whites
- Asthma-related mortality rates are lower among Mexican-Americans than among non-Latino whites and non-Latino blacks

➤ Domestic violence

➤ Prevalence rates among Latinos are *lower* for the following:
- Psychiatric disorders
- Overall rates of cancer
- Cardiovascular death rates
- Infant and maternal mortality

Summary of Obstacles to Health Care Delivery and Risk Factors for Disease in Latinos

Obstacles to Health Care Delivery

- Immigrants granted legal resident status cannot receive Medicaid until after 5 years' residence
- Fear of INS involvement

Women
- Embarrassment about sexual matters may delay or prevent access to gynecologic care; low rate of Pap smears
- Child care and responsibilities toward family may make attending to personal health a low priority

Men
- Issues of masculinity (e.g., toleration of pain) may delay or discourage access to health care
  - ➤ Concerns about sexual side effects of medication
  - ➤ Less likely to report homosexual practices
- Values regarding self-sufficiency delay or discourage access to health care
- Distrust regarding medical treatments or products having "artificial" origins
- Fatalism
- Lack of insurance coverage even among employed, non-poor Latinos
- Limited Medicaid access
- Language barriers (see Summary Box on Communication Issues in Caring for Latinos on page 90)
- Low education levels and literacy rates
- Perceived or real discrimination and prejudice
- Lack of access to automobile, particularly in rural areas or in cities with more limited public transportation systems (e.g., Los Angeles)
- Missing work to meet doctor appointments may not be feasible

Health Risk Factors

- Men are less likely to use condoms; women may have difficulty negotiating condom use with partner.
- Injection drug use is more common; however, Latinos are less likely to use illicit drugs than non-Latino whites.
- Puerto Ricans are more likely to smoke than other Latino groups.
- Mexican-Americans diets have higher cholesterol and total fat than diets of other Latino groups.

Summary of Communication Issues in Caring for Latinos

Limited English Language Proficiency

➤ Rates of limited English language proficiency are highest in first-generation immigrants.

➤ Limited English language proficiency creates health care problems for Latino patients:
  • Less satisfaction with doctor-patient interaction
  • Fewer doctor visits
  • Less likely to receive a follow-up appointment
  • Poorer health outcomes

➤ Provide bilingual written materials (e.g., signage, posters, patient education materials).

➤ Provide bilingual telephone systems.

➤ Provide professional medical interpreter services because 1) interpreters are trained to translate medical terminology and 2) physicians tend to overestimate their foreign-language proficiency.
  • Family members or friends of the patient should not be used as interpreters because of issues of confidentially.
  • Latino patients may not ask for interpreters out of respect for the physician, so interpreter services should be offered.

➤ Second-generation Latinos are likely to be bilingual.

Nonverbal Communication and Family Relationships

➤ Latinos may make less eye contact than non-Latino whites.

➤ Nonverbal signs of personal warmth (e.g., smiles, handshakes) are highly valued by Latinos.

➤ Because Latinos tend to value trust and warm personal relationships, they may prefer health care providers who take a personal interest in their lives; however, use formal address (Mr/Mrs; Señor/Señora), especially with older patients, and wear professional attire.

➤ Involve family members, but bear in mind that they may wish to shield the patient from bad news; there may be possible conflicts with informed consent policies.

REFERENCES

1. Ramirez RR. The Hispanic Population in the United States, March 1999. Washington, DC: Department of Commerce, Economics and Statistics Administration, Bureau of the Census; 2000; PPL-124.

2. Schur CL, Feldman J. Running in place: how job characteristics, immigrant status, and family structure keep Hispanics uninsured. New York: The Commonwealth Fund; May 2001.

3. History of Cuba. Brittanica.com and Encyclopaedia Britannica; 1999-2000.

4. History of the Dominican Republic. Brittanica.com and Encyclopaedia Britannica; 1999-2000.

5. Hajat A, Lucas JB, Kington R. Health outcomes among Hispanic subgroups: data from the National Health Interview Study, 1992-5. Washington, DC: Centers for Disease Control and National Center for Health Statistics, DHHS Publication (PHS) 2000-1934, Series 21, No. 56 0-0039; January 2000.

6. Adult Literacy in America—1992. Prepared by the Educational Testing Service. Washington, DC: Department of Education, National Center for Education Statistics, National Adult Literacy Survey; 1992.

7. Working Without Benefits: The Health Insurance Crisis Confronting Hispanic Americans. Task Force on the Future of Health Insurance for Working Americans. New York: The Commonwealth Fund; March 2000.

8. Marin BV, Tschann JM, Gomez CA, Kegeles SM. Acculturation and gender differences in sexual attitudes and behaviors: Hispanic vs. non-Hispanic white adults. Am J Public Health. 1993;83:1759-61.

9. Sandman D, Simantov E, An C. Out of Touch: American Men and the Health Care System. New York: The Commonwealth Fund; March 2000.

10. Collins KS, Hall A, Neuhaus C. US Minority Health: A Chartbook. New York: The Commonwealth Fund; 1999.

11. Molina CW, Aguirre-Molina M, eds. Latino Health in the United States: A Growing Challenge. Washington, DC: American Public Health Association; 1994.

12. Worsley P. Non-Western medical systems. Ann Rev Anthropology. 1982;11:319.

12a. Liebowitz MR, Salman E, Jusino CM, et al. Ataque de nervios and panic disorder. Am J Psychiatry. 1994;151:871-5.

13. Graham JS. Mexican-American herbal remedies: an evaluation. Herbalgram. 31 July 1994, No. 31, pp 34-6; available via AMED database (Allied and Complementary Medicine, Ovid Technologies).

14. Zayas LH, Ozuah PO. Mercury use in espiritismo: a survey of botanicas. Am J Pub Health. 1996;86:111-2.

15. Oman D, Red D. Religion and mortality among the community-dwelling elderly. Am J Public Health. 1998;88:1469-75.

16. Norris J, Harnack L, Carmichael S, et al. US trends in nutrient intake: the 1987 and 1992 National Health Interview Surveys. Am J Public Health. 1997;87:740-6.

17. Kuczmarski MF, Kuczmarski R, Jajjar M. Food usage among Mexican-American, Cuban, and Puerto Rican adults: findings from the Hispanic HANES. Nutrition Today. 1996;30: 30-7.

18. Loria CM, Bush TL, Carroll MD, et al. Macronutrient intakes among adult Hispanics: a comparison of Mexican Americans, Cuban Americans and mainland Puerto Ricans. Am J Public Health. 1995;85:684-9.

19. Guendelman S, Abrams B. Dietary intake among Mexican American women: generational differences and a comparison with white non-Hispanic women. Am J Public Health. 1995;85:20-5.

20. Hajat A, et al. Health Outcomes among Hispanic subgroups: data from the National Health Interview Study, 1992-5. Washington, DC: Department of Health and Human Services, Centers for Disease Control, National Center for Health Statistics; Number 310, 25 February 2000.

21. Kington RS, Smith JP. Socioeconomic status and racial and ethnic differences in functional status associated with chronic diseases. Am J Public Health. 1997;87:805-10.

22. Abraido-Lanza AF, Dohrenwend BP, Ng-Mak DS, Turner JB. The Latino mortality paradox: a test of the "salmon bias" and healthy migrant hypotheses. Am J Public Health. 1999;8:1543-8.

23. Ventura SJ, et al. Trends in Pregnancies and Pregnancy Rates by Outcome: Estimates for the United States, 1979-96. Division of Vital Statistics, DHHS Publication (PHS) 2000-1934, Series 21, No. 56, 0-0039; January 2000.

24. Bolen JC, Rhodes L, Powell-Griner EE, et al. State-Specific Prevalence of Selected Health Behaviors by Race and Ethnicity. Division of Adult and Community Health, National Center for Chronic Disease Prevention and Health Promotion, Behavioral Risk Factor Surveillance System; 1997.

25. Suarez L. Pap smear and mammogram screening in Mexican American women: the effects of acculturation. Am J Public Health. 1994;84:742-6.

26. Herbert R, Landrigan PJ. Work-related death: a continuing epidemic. Am J Public Health. 2000;90:541-5.

27. Maizlish N, Rudolph L. California adults with elevated blood levels, 1987 through 1990. Am J Public Health. 1993;83:402-5.

28. Highway Safety Needs of US Hispanic Communities: Issues and Strategies. Washington, DC: National Highway Traffic Safety Administration; DOT HS 808 373; available from the NHTSA Web site.

29. Mokdad AH, Serdula MK, Dietx WH, et al. The spread of the obesity epidemic in the United States, 1991-1998. JAMA. 1999;282:1519-22.

30. Brownson RC, Eyler AA, King AC, et al. Patterns and correlates of physical activity among US women 40 years and older. Am J Public Health. 2000;90:264-70.

31. Sowers JR. Modest weight gain and the development of diabetes: another perspective. Ann Intern Med. 1995;122:548-9.

32. Harris MI. Medical care for patients with diabetes: epidemiologic aspects. Ann Intern Med. 1996;124:117-22.

33. Black SA, Ray LA, Markides KS. The prevalence and health burden of self-reported diabetes in older Mexican Americans: findings from the Hispanic Established Populations for Epidemiologic Studies of the Elderly. Am J Public Health. 1999;89:546-52.

34. Burke JP, Williams K, Gaskill SP, et al. Rapid rise in the incidence of type 2 diabetes from 1987 to 1996: results from the San Antonio Heart Study. Arch Intern Med. 1999;159:1450-6.

35. Crespo CJ, Loria CM, Burt VL. Hypertension and other cardiovascular disease risk factors among Mexican Americans, Cuban Americans, and Puerto Ricans from the Hispanic Health and Nutrition Examination Survey. Public Health Rep. 1996;111:7-10.

36. Liao Y, Coper RS, Cao G, et al. Mortality from coronary heart disease and cardiovascular disease among adult US Hispanics: findings from the National Health Interview Survey (1986 to 1994). J Am Coll Cardiol. 1997;30:1200-5.

37. Carlisle DM, Leake BD, Shapiro MF. Racial and ethnic disparities in the use of cardio-vascular procedures: associations with type of health insurance. Am J Public Health. 1997:87:263-7.

38. Norris SL, DeGuzman M, Sobel E, et al. Risk factors and mortality among black, Caucasian and Latino women with acute myocardial infarction. Am Heart J. 1993;126:1312-9.

39. Hewitt M, Simone JV, eds. Ensuring Quality Cancer Care. National Cancer Policy Board, Institute of Medicine and National Research Council; 1999.

40. Cleeland CS, Gonin R, Baez L, et al. Pain and treatment of pain in minority patients with cancer. The Eastern Cooperative Group Minority Outpatient Pain Study. Ann Intern Med. 1997;127:813-6.

41. Klevens RM, Diaz T, Fleming PL, et al. Trends in AIDS among Hispanics in the United States, 1991-1996. Am J Public Health. 1999;89:1104-6.

42. Moore RD, Stanton D, Gopalan R, Chaisson RE. Racial differences in the use of drug therapy for HIV disease in an urban community. N Engl J Med. 1994;330:763-8.

43. Laine C, Newshaffer CJ, Zhang D, et al. Adherence to antiretroviral therapy by pregnant women infected with human immunodeficiency virus: a pharmacy claims-based analysis. Obstet Gynecol. 2000;95:167-73.

44. Sikkema KJ, Heckman TG, Kelly JA, et al. HIV risk behaviors among women living in low-income, inner-city housing developments. Am J Public Health. 1996;86:1123-8.

45. Sikkema KJ, Kelly JA, Winett RA, et al. Outcomes of a randomized community-level HIV prevention intervention for women living in 18 low-income housing developments. Am J Public Health. 2000;90:57-63.

46. Recommendations for prevention and control of hepatitis C virus (HCV) infection and HCV-related chronic disease. MMWR. 1998;47:1-39.

47. Alderete E, Vega WA, Kolody B, Aguilar-Gaxiola S. Lifetime prevalence of and risk factors for psychiatric disorders among Mexican migrant farmworkers in California. Am J Public Health. 2000;90:608-14.

48. Padgett DK, Patrick C, Burns BJ, Schlesinger JH. Ethnicity and the use of outpatient mental health services in a national insured population. Am J Public Health. 1994;84: 222-6.

49. Homa DM, Mannino DM, Lara M. Asthma mortality in U.S. Hispanics of Mexican, Puerto Rican, and Cuban heritage, 1990-1995. Am J Respir Crit Care Med. 2000:161; 504-9.

50. Ledogar RJ, Penchaszadeh C, Garden CI, Acosta LG. Asthma and Latino cultures: different prevalence reported among groups sharing the same environment. Am J Public Health. 2000;90:929-35.

51. Lara M, Allen F, Lange L. Physician perceptions of barriers to care for inner-city Latino children with asthma. J Health Care Poor Underserved. 1999;10:27-44.

52. Detailed Language Spoken at Home and Ability to Speak English for Persons 5 Years and Over: The 50 Languages with the Greatest Number of Speakers. 1990 U.S. Census; available at http://www.census.gov/population/socdemo/language/table5.txt.

53. Collins KS, Hughes DL, Doty MM, et al. Diverse Communities, Common Concerns: Assessing Health Care Quality for Minority Americans. New York: The Commonwealth Fund; March 2002.

54. Carrasquillo O, Orav EJ, Brennan TA, Burstin HR. Impact of language barriers on patient satisfaction in an emergency department. J Gen Intern Med. 1999;14:82-7.

55. Sarver J, Baker DW. Effect of language barriers on follow-up appointments after an emergency department visit. J Gen Intern Med. 2000;15:256-64.

56. Waxman MA, Levitt MA. Are diagnostic testing and admission rates higher in non-English-speaking versus English-speaking patients in the emergency department? Ann Emerg Med. 2000;36:456-61.

57. Hampers LC, Cha S, Gutglass DJ, et al. Language barriers and resource utilization in a pediatric emergency department. Pediatrics. 1999;103:1253-6.

58. Todd KH, Lee T, Hoffman JR. The effect of ethnicity on physician estimates of pain severity in patients with isolated extremity trauma. JAMA. 1994;274:925-8.

4

Care of American Indians and Alaska Natives

CHRISTINE MAKOSKY DALEY, MA, SM
SEAN M. DALEY, MA

Ever since the arrival of Columbus in the New World in 1492 Indians have been misrepresented and misunderstood by the non-Indian world.[1] The term *Indian* itself is a misnomer. The naming of the residents of the Americas as *Indians*, or *los Indios* as Columbus called them, came from his belief that he had landed in or near the East Indies. Even after his error was realized, the term remained. The French word *Indien*, the German *Indianer*, and the English *Indian* are all derivatives of the original Spanish term (1).

From the beginning, *Indian* was used as a blanket term, a convenient way to identify any member of any Nation. Contrary to common belief, however, there was no homogeneous culture or single language among the residents of America:

> The residents of the Americas were by modern estimates divided into at least two thousand cultures and more societies, practiced a multiplicity of customs and lifestyles, held an enormous variety of values and beliefs, spoke numerous languages mutually unintelligible to the many speakers, and did not conceive of themselves as a single people (1).

Today the term *Indian* remains in general use. It allows the classification of all Natives under one heading without having to consider and individually itemize the social and cultural diversity found among the many Native nations (e.g., Cheyenne, Tlingit, Hopi).

---

[1] The term *Indian* is used throughout this chapter to refer to the people of the First Nations of the Americas, because it has been the experience of the authors that this term is preferred by First Nations peoples.

The United States contains 558 federally recognized Indian nations and Alaska Native villages and 2.5 million individuals claiming Indian or Alaska Native ancestry (2). Native Hawaiians are not included in these figures because they are not "Native Americans", or "American Indians", according to federal government definitions. Who is and who is not an Indian is not always an easy question to answer:

> Not all individuals claiming to be Indian "look Indian", nor were many born into tribal environments. Many are not tribally enrolled, and others who claim to be Indian are not Indian at all. Some Indians who appear Caucasian or black go back and forth assuming Indian, white, and black identities, while others who have lived most of their lives as non-Indians decide to "become Indians" at a later age. Some individuals are Indian by virtue of biological connection but know little about their cultural mores because of lack of interest, because there was no one to teach them, or because it was not (or is not) socially or economically profitable to pursue an Indian identity due to the time period, location, and degree of racism, prejudice, and stereotypes (3).

The federal government acknowledges only officially recognized tribes as Indian. To be federally recognized, an Indian nation must petition the Branch of Acknowledgement and Research of the Bureau of Indian Affairs and meet certain criteria, such as having signed a treaty with the United States government. Groups that are federally recognized receive the "perks" that many non-Indians think of as "breaks" or "benefits" for being Indian, such as medical aid from the Indian Health Service (IHS), exemption from certain taxes, and permission to run gaming facilities. Groups that are not federally recognized may be legally recognized by the state in which they reside and receive limited benefits.

Each Indian group has its own rules for membership. For example, according to present-day Navajo law, membership in the Navajo Nation requires that a person be at least one-quarter Navajo and not a member of any other Indian tribe (4).

Indian-White Relations

Relations between Indians and whites have generally been poor. Many Indian-white interactions have been marked by white ethnocentrism, or the belief that white Euro-American cultural practices are superior to

Indian cultures and lifeways. The post-Contact (after Columbus's arrival) history of the Western hemisphere is marked by disease, colonialism, and genocide. Discussed here are a few areas of Indian-white relations that have been problematic and that have intensified the distrust that Indians have for whites and white medicine.

White Diseases in the New World

Much of the first contact Native peoples in the Americas had with Europeans came through disease, particularly smallpox, though measles and typhus also played a large role in the devastation of the Native population. One of the earliest recorded smallpox outbreaks in the New World was in the Aztec capital of Tenochtitlan (the present-day Mexico City), a city of approximately 200,000 to 250,000 inhabitants. When Cortez attacked the city in 1520, he had approximately 1200 men; after the fighting only 300 remained. Cortez retreated but returned a year later with 600 reinforcements and a small relief force, one member of which was carrying the smallpox virus. Because of previous exposure to the disease, Cortez's troops were virtually unaffected. The unexposed Aztecs, however, were soon overcome by the virus; almost all were infected, one-third fatally. Cortez won an easy victory (5,6).

Over the following centuries smallpox spread throughout the New World, leaving devastation in its path. Between 1837 and 1840, an epidemic swept across the Great Plains, killing approximately 40,000 Blackfoot and all but exterminating the Mandan. After reaching Alaska it killed 60% of the Alaska Native population. Most of the spread of smallpox (and other infectious diseases) came through traders who moved across the continent before the settlers. Many Natives now claim that in the 1800s the federal government handed out blankets infested with the virus, knowing Indians had no resistance to the disease. It can at least be said that exposure to European diseases left many Natives throughout the Americas more than distrustful of whites and their medicine.

Forced Assimilation

The Court of Indian Offenses

European explorers, missionaries, and government officials usually tried to change Indian cultural practices. When the United States became a sovereign nation, it continued the practice of trying to stamp out Indian identity and culture and replace them with those of the white Christian majority.

The Court of Indian Offenses was established in 1883 at the suggestion of Henry M. Teller, Secretary of the Interior. Teller's goal was to eliminate certain traditional Indian practices that he, and most Americans, viewed as immoral and savage. These practices, they believed, only hindered the Indian's climb up the ladder of civilization. Minor offenses would also be suitably punished (7).

On the reservations, Indian agents, government officials, and missionaries were quick to implement and enforce the codes established by the Court. For example, an Indian who engaged in tribal dances faced withholding of rations or imprisonment for 10 days for a first offense, and an Indian who practiced as medicine man faced imprisonment for 10 to 30 days (8).

Indian Boarding Schools

There were other ways the federal government used laws and policies to further its goal of assimilating Indians. Indian boarding schools, prominent in the late 1800s and early 1900s, were federally funded institutions that taught Indian children how to live properly (i.e., by white standards). Indian children were taken away from their families and reservations and sent to these schools, often hundreds of miles away. Many graduates of Indian boarding schools forgot their Native languages, religious traditions, and ways of life.

The Termination Era

The Termination Era is roughly defined as the years between 1945 and 1962. During this time the position of the federal government was that most of the problems facing Indians, such as poor housing and sanitation, lack of jobs, and poverty, could be eliminated if tribal groups were dissolved and if tribal lands and resources were liquidated. The Termination Era had three major components:

1. In 1953, House Concurrent Resolution 108 (HCR 108) declared it to be the policy of the United States to abolish federal supervision over Indian tribes as soon as possible and to subject Indians to the same laws, privileges, and responsibilities as other

American citizens (7). Thus the unique relationship between the tribes and the federal government was to be severed.

2. As a consequence of HCR 108, Public Law 280 (PL 280), also adapted in 1953, transferred substantial federal civil and criminal jurisdiction regarding Indian matters to state governments in certain states with high Indian populations.

3. The physical relocation of Indians from reservations to cities was to be encouraged. This component of Termination, commonly referred to as Relocation, promised Indians good-paying jobs and places to live if they voluntarily left their reservations for urban areas. However, when many Relocation participants arrived in the cities, there were no jobs or housing waiting for them. Of those who did manage to obtain jobs and housing, approximately 30% left the Relocation program and returned to the reservation within 12 months; this percentage rose during the second year.[2]

Terminated tribes faced social, economic, and political upheaval on both the community and personal levels. For example, two years after the Klamath of Oregon were terminated, Klamath men no longer worked at the once tribally owned mills. Alcoholism and family problems rose markedly (9). Overall, during the Termination Era, 100 tribes were terminated, approximately 12,000 individuals lost tribal affiliations, and approximately 2.5 million acres of Indian land were lost (4). Although the federal government never officially abandoned Termination policies, they are no longer actively pursued. Most of the terminated tribes have had their federal recognition restored, but a few are still waiting for reinstatement.

The 21st Century

Today, Indians do not possess the numbers, financial resources, or political clout to be a major force in the United States. Indians do have influence on a few local or state governments (e.g., in Arizona and Washington), but their power is usually tenuous and often challenged.

---

[2] Robert Bee, personal communication, 1999. Relocation programs are still used by the federal government. Currently they are referred to as Employment Assistance Programs.

Medicine, Illness, and Religion

Attributes of a Colonial System

The expropriation, colonization, and settlement of Indian lands by white soldiers and pioneers have necessarily affected the way Indians view the modern world. According to Robert Bee (personal communication, 1999), there are three attributes of a colonial system:

1. *Economic Exploitation*—Natives are exploited for cheap labor, and their land is exploited for its natural resources.

2. *Political Domination*—Natives are disarmed, and their ability to wage war is eliminated. They no longer have the power to govern themselves but must follow the laws and dictates of the colonizer.

3. *Cultural Domination*—Traditional religions and ceremonies are banned, and Native children are instructed in the colonizer's ways and culture. The colonizer seeks to assimilate Natives by re-placing their mores, teachings, and beliefs by those of the new ruling class.

To these three, a fourth attribute of colonization can provisionally be added:

4. *Medical Domination*—Under most, if not all, colonial systems, indigenous peoples are not allowed to continue traditional med-icinal practices. Access is restricted to needed medicinal materi-als (i.e., plants, animals); traditional healers are no longer able to practice medicine; and techniques too closely aligned with Native religious practices are outlawed. These traditional healing systems are then replaced by the dominant healing system of the colonizer—in the case of Native North Americans, by biomedi-cine. Thus, in the minds of many Indians, biomedicine is an ex-tension of colonialism.

Numbers 1 to 3 above have been discussed briefly in the section on Indian-White Relations. This section looks at Indian attitudes concerning science and medicine, illness and healing, and, necessarily, religion. Many

Indians believe that Western science does not, as is claimed by its disciples, involve discovering and examining basic truths about the natural world, but rather is a Eurocentric teaching imposed by a more powerful culture on a weaker one. Deloria claims that in mainstream American society scientists have assumed the role of religious leaders; that is, people expect them to answer their fundamental questions about life and death (10). It is the view of many Indians that, in fact, scientists possess no "true" knowledge about the world and the deeper questions of existence and mortality.

Intertribalism and Pan-Indianism

Just as there are similarities between the various cultures and nations in Western Europe, so too for the many Indian nations in the United States. *Intertribalism*, or the exchanging of traits between different Indian nations (11), and *pan-Indianism*, or a general sense of Indian cultural identity that unites members of different Indian nations (12), are both terms commonly used to refer to the similarities between Indian nations. For example, because many Indian nations use feathers from eagles, hawks, and turkeys in religious ceremonies, feathers have become an inter-tribal, or pan-Indian, symbol.

For convenience, then, the non-Western world-views discussed below can be taken as generally representative of all Indian nations. It must be kept in mind, however, that different beliefs exist between tribes and that no single tribe can represent all facets of Indian culture.

World-Views

World-view can be defined as how a group of people (or a culture) views the cosmos and one's place in it, the causes of events, moral and ethical issues, and so on. Many components make up one's world-view, but most include religion and attitudes to medicine and healing. It is nearly impossible to separate religion from medicine in many cultures, including those of Native North Americans, whereas other cultures have a thick dividing line between them. Therefore to understand a people's ethnomedical beliefs it is necessary to understand their world-view.

Medicine, religion, and magic are closely related in a *personalistic system*. Personalistic systems have multiple levels of causality (often involving the spirit world). Illness is considered beyond the control of the patient, and positive actions (often related to religious practices) can be used as prevention. A powerful active agent (often supernatural) causes illness, and illness in turn is seen as a special case of misfortune, again often tied to the spirit world or other supernatural forces. In a *naturalistic system,* on the other hand, medicine is largely unrelated to religion and magic; causality is often on a single level and rarely involves the spirit world. Illness is usually caused by some kind of equilibrium loss (e.g., a pathogen taking over the host). Prevention is best practiced by avoidance of certain actions or things. Much of the responsibility for illness and prevention resides within the patient himself or herself (13). Though there is overlap between these two systems, their major difference is the influence of religion. If biomedical ideas could be explained using more personalistic terms, however, the gap between the two systems may at least be partially narrowed.

When world-views are examined cross-culturally, two major schools of thought emerge: Western and non-Western. The Western world-view focuses on Eurocentric ideas and the strong influence of the Judeo-Christian tradition. Most of Europe, North America, and Australia subscribe to this world-view, at least since the time of Contact. Most of the rest of the world and the colonized peoples of North America and Australia, on the other hand, subscribe to a non-Western world-view. According to Robert Bee (personal communication, 2000), there are eight tenets of the non-Western world-view:

1. There is no relevant difference between the natural and the supernatural; these concepts are mixed and work together. Indian religions generally do not draw a clear dividing line between this world (the physical world, the natural world) and the spirit world. For instance, many Indian nations (e.g., Iroquois, Cherokee, Yaqui, Navajo) have masked dancers during their ceremonies. These masked dancers, most often men, dress as certain spirits or deities. While dressed in this manner, the dancers are imbued with the powers and qualities of the spirits or deities being imitated. To show disrespect to a masked dancer would be the same as showing disrespect to the spirit or deity being imitated.

2. There is fundamental equality between human beings and their environment. Humans are not considered "higher" than other parts of the natural environment (e.g., plants, animals); rather, all are part of nature and depend on it for survival. Most Judeo-Christian doctrines teach that man is superior to nature and that man is to control and shape nature as he pleases. This notion is the basis for many Euro-American agricultural practices and land tenure and ownership patterns. However, most Indian nations do not follow such strict separation between man and the environment. For example, in an Indian nation in the Southwest an elder needs plants for medicinal or ceremonial purposes. Once a plant is located, the elder sings a traditional song, makes an offering of a sacred stone or other object, recites a prayer, and walks around the plant sunwise (clockwise). The plants are picked only when needed and only in the amount necessary. Plants of the same species are then gathered in the same vicinity. If these things are not done, the plant will be offended and not work properly as a medicine or in the ceremony.

3. There is a personalized and dynamic interaction between humans, spirits, nature, and power. This relationship can be seen as an extension of human social relationships. Among the Lakota, for example, often erroneously referred to as the Sioux, exists the *Wanagi yuhapi,* or Ghost-Keeping Ceremony. The Lakota believe that when a person dies, his or her spirit travels along the "ghost road" until it is met by an old woman. The old woman decides if the spirit will be allowed to travel on to the hereafter and live with his or her relatives already there or will be ordered back to the earth where it will live as an evil ghost (14). However, the family of the deceased may elect to keep his or her spirit with them for a time. In the Ghost-Keeping Ceremony a piece of the deceased, such as a lock of hair, is bound up in a spirit bundle and treated as if it were alive for one year. After the year has passed, at a great feast the spirit is fed for the last time and then released (15).

4. Power is what makes the system dynamic. If one part of the system (such as a person) wishes to make the system work to his or her benefit, he or she must have and use power. Among the Apache of Arizona, for instance, power (*diyi*) plays an important role in religious and medical thought. According to Basso, Apaches are specific as to what power does or can do, but they are uneasy explaining what power is (16). Apaches state that power possesses the attribute of holiness; the Apache live in a world where everything has power (17). Apaches are capable of acquiring power through different means and using and manipulating it through ritual. However, there can be negative consequences for those who disrespect power.

5. Rituals are used to harness and manipulate power. Ordinarily, rituals must be performed correctly or they will not be successful. Once a person has built up power through the use of rituals or by following specific cultural rules, he or she can use this power to do good or evil. A fetish is generally a small carved figure, usually representing a bird, animal, or spirit, that is believed to have power. It is believed that a spirit resides in the object, as with Zuni hunting fetishes, which are said to be the shrunken images of great animal gods that control hunting and war. The hunter or warrior prays directly to the fetish and either breathes on it or breathes from it (18). If this ritual is performed correctly, he should receive aid and protection from the spirit.

6. Nothing happens by "chance" but through the manipulation of power. All events, good or evil, occur because some part of the system wanted them to happen that way. Many Indian cultures attribute illness and bad luck to witchcraft, ghosts, and taboo violations. A stubbed toe may not be as simple as a stubbed toe; there is probably some greater reason as to why this happened. According to traditional Hopi belief, for example, illnesses, crop failure, bad behavior, and other undesirable happenings are usually the result of witchcraft (19).

7. Time is cyclical, like the seasons. Western cultures, on the other hand, often see time in a linear fashion, progressing towards some goal or ultimate end. Most Indian cultures view time and its progression differently than do Western cultures. Rather than being a straight line comprising past, present, and future, time is seen more as a coiled spring that has been expanded. Yes, time does progress and there is a past, a present, and a future; however, events that occurred in the past may still affect man, individually and collectively, in the present and in the future, on physical, mental, emotional, and spiritual levels. The Navajo believe that once an event has taken place its effects may be repeated at any future time; for instance, occurrences in the Underworlds (Navajo oral history teaches that they once lived in four subterranean worlds below this, the fifth world) still affect this world and man (20). A Navajo may suffer from an illness because of a parental taboo violation years before his or her birth.

8. All tenets of world-view rest on a series of origin narratives. Each culture has a unique origin narrative that explains how humans were created, what causes things to happen, the difference between right and wrong, and other prescribed rules. The prevailing scientific theory of Indian origins is the Bering Strait hypothesis. According to this theory, between 28,000 and 12,000 years ago the ancestors of today's Indians (Paleo-Indians or Paleo-Siberians), following large herds of grazing animals, crossed an expansive area of exposed land (the Bering Land Bridge) that connected northeastern Asia to western Alaska during the last Ice Age and began spreading throughout the Americas (19).

Indians, however, do not mention the Bering Strait hypothesis when explaining their origins; they have their own tribal beliefs. For example, according to the Kiowa, a southern Plains nation presently found in Oklahoma, they

> . . .came one by one into the world through a hollow log. They were many more than now, but not all of them got out. There was a woman whose body was swollen up with child, and she got stuck in the log. After that, no one could get through, and that is why the Kiowas are small in number. They looked all around and saw the world. It made them glad to see so many things. They called themselves *Kwuda,* "coming out" (21).

Sebastian LeBeau, a Lakota and the Cheyenne River Sioux Repatriation Officer, has stated:

> We never asked science to make a determination as to our origins. We know where we came from. We are descendants of the Buffalo people. . .If non-Indians choose to believe they evolved from an ape so be it. I have yet to come across five Lakotas who believe in science and in evolution" (22).

To summarize, medicine and healing are integrated more clearly with religion in non-Western than in Western cultures. Power, as the dynamic element, both causes and cures illness when manipulated in different ways and there is necessarily more interaction with nature and the spirit world. As such, it is impossible to cure a person, part of the natural world, without addressing spiritual issues. In Western cultures, medicine often ignores the spiritual aspects of health, making it difficult for a person with a non-Western world-view (e.g., American Indians and Alaska Natives) to accept "cure" through Western medicine.

Wellness and Unwellness

The Native American Research and Training Center at the University of Arizona has listed ten attributes of wellness and unwellness that apply to most Indian nations (Table 4-1).[3] Although it is possible to discuss pan-Indian beliefs, these beliefs present only a partial picture. With over 550 nations, not all will subscribe to all beliefs and all will have some beliefs that are unique to themselves. Navajo or Diné, as they call themselves, concepts of wellness and unwellness are discussed in Box 4-1.

---

[3] The terms *wellness* and *unwellness* are used instead of *ill, illness, sick,* or *sickness.* The former terms tend to be more encompassing, including physical, mental, emotional, and spiritual ailments, than the latter. In addition, the latter terms are more often associated with Western or biomedical health systems.

Table 4-1 American Indian Attributes of Wellness and Unwellness
1. There is a Supreme Creator.
2. Humans have a body, mind, and spirit.
3. All things, living or not, have a spirit.
4. The spirit existed before the physical body and will exist after the death of the physical body.
5. Illness affects the body, mind, and spirit.
6. Wellness is the harmony of body, mind, and spirit.
7. Unwellness is the disharmony of body, mind, and spirit.
8. Natural illness exists (e.g., taboo violation).
9. Unnatural illness exists (e.g., witchcraft).
10. We ourselves are responsible for our health.

From American Indian Conceptions of Wellness and Unwellness. Tucson, Arizona: Native American Research and Training Center; 1997; with permission.

The Indian Health Service (IHS)

Based on the more than 350 treaties signed between the United States government and various Indian nations between the late 1700s and the late 1800s, members of federally recognized tribes are guaranteed participation in federal health care programs. Health care is provided through the Indian Health Service (IHS), originally part of the Bureau of Indian Affairs (BIA) and now part of the Department of Health and Human Services (DHHS). In 1954, the Division of Health set four priorities (2):

1. To assemble a competent health staff
2. To establish adequate facilities
3. To initiate extensive curative treatment for those seriously ill
4. To develop a full-scale prevention program aimed at reducing excessive rates of illness and early death from preventable diseases and conditions

The Indian Self-Determination and Education Assistance Act of 1975 expanded IHS policy by giving tribes the ability to staff and manage IHS programs in their communities if they so chose. As a result, many Native

Box 4-1   Navajo Religion and Medicine

In most Indian nations, the line between religion and medicine is a thin one, if it exists at all. This holds true for the Navajo Nation. According to Kluckhohn and Leighton (Kluckhohn C, Leighton D. The Navaho, rev. ed. Garden City, New York: Doubleday; 1962), at first glance the Navajo religion appears to be one of fear, not of belief.* Though an overstatement, there are certainly "Do's" and "Don't's" based on traditional conceptions of the universe and the Navajo's place in it.

What is the Navajo world-view? One reference states that its building blocks are activity, creativity, control, balance, order, and beauty (Witherspoon G. Language and Art in the Navajo Universe. Ann Arbor: University of Michigan Press; 1979). Another claims that for Navajos there are no forces, no equilibriums, no dynamisms, no processes; there are only people, great people, and Holy People (Luckert KW. Coyoteway: A Navajo Holyway Healing Ceremonial. Tucson/Flagstaff: University of Arizona Press and Museum of Northern Arizona Press; 1972). Both interpretations have been criticized by Navajo and non-Navajo alike. In the authors' experience there is a definite emphasis by the Navajo on order, harmony, and beauty, yet these concepts are often closely connected to various religious figures (e.g., healers, singers, deities) and their activities.

One of the metaphysical premises of the Navajo world-view is that of *hozho* and *hochoo* (also spelled *hochxo*). *Hozho* is often defined as beauty or harmony, *hochoo* as ugliness or disharmony. This premise is not a simple, dualistic notion (e.g., good versus evil) but is more complicated. According to Farella, the origin of the Navajo can be described in terms of the creation of wholes that are pairings of opposites or complements. One cannot define beauty unless there is ugliness with which to contrast it; eliminate one and the other is eliminated as well (Farella JR. The Main Stalk: A Synthesis of Navajo Philosophy. Tucson: University of Arizona Press; 1984). In addition, *hozho* and *hochoo* are ongoing processes, both being constantly created and destroyed.

Hozho and *hochoo* are essential to the Navajo conception of the "good life". Many Navajo say they want to "walk in beauty", meaning that they want to live a good, productive, and healthy life, a life of *hozho*. This may not always be possible, however, for a number of reasons, and then one becomes unwell (*hochoo*). *Hochoo* may be brought about accidentally or willfully. An obvious way in which *hochoo* can occur is by leading an out-of-control life (e.g., excessive drinking,

---

* Although there exists no word for "religion" in the Navajo language; the closest equivalent being *nahaga* ("a ceremony is taking place"), and use of the word "religion" is often deemed problematic, the word is used here for ease and simplicity.

(Cont'd.)

Box 4-1 (continued)

excessive sex). Of course, anyone leading such a life, Navajo or non-Navajo, runs the risk of becoming ill or unwell. From a Navajo's point of view, however, lack of control is disharmonious on a spiritual level as well. Disharmony is *hochoo; hochoo* is unwellness. Other things, more particular to the Navajo, may bring about *hochoo;* for example, a sandpainting must be created by a singer (erroneously called a "medicine man") in a clockwise manner starting in the east; if it is created in any other direction, it will cause evil and illness (Bulow E. Navajo Taboos. Gallup, New Mexico: Buffalo Medicine Books; 1991).

Kluckhohn's *Navaho Witchcraft* was the first, and is still one of the few, thorough studies of the subject (Kluckhohn C. Navaho Witchcraft. Papers of the Peabody Museum of American Archaeology and Ethnology. Harvard University; 1944). According to Kluckhohn, witchcraft is one of the most hideous activities in which a Navajo can partake. The witch's goal is to bring about *hochoo.* To take the example above: witches create sandpaintings in a counter-clockwise fashion, intentionally bringing about evil and illness. Witches are also associated with death and incest, two very dangerous things, because they are associated with the underworlds where unwellness originated (Franciscan Fathers: An Ethnological Dictionary of the Navaho Language. St. Michaels, Arizona: Navajo Indian Missions; 1910).

If a Navajo becomes unwell, one of several ceremonies, or a "sing" in Navajo parlance, must be performed. The particular ceremony employed depends upon the nature of the unwellness. For example, a Coyoteway (a division of the Evilway ceremonials) may be called for in the case of incest (Luckert, *op. cit.*), while an Excessway or Prostitutionway may be called upon to combat Moth Madness, the ill effects of Love Magic (Kluckhohn and Leighton, *op. cit.;* Levy JE, Neutra R, Parker D. Hand Trembling, Frenzy Witchcraft, and Moth Madness. Tucson: University of Arizona Press; 1987). Navajo conceptions of wellness and unwellness are directly related to the fundamental premises of *hozho* and *hochoo.* Excess, taboo violations, and witchcraft bring about disharmony, lack of control—*hochoo.* A sing is needed to restore the harmony and balance—*hozho.*

Within Navajo medicine, plants play a large role. Herbs have both ceremonial and medicinal uses. Singers, who normally collect the plants for ceremonies, generally have knowledge of about 100 plant varieties. Herbalists know the most about plants; they are learned in over 300 varieties and their uses. Besides these two specialists, most households have at least one person with

Box 4-1 (continued)

some botanical knowledge who gathers plants for home remedies. These plants are part of the largest family within the Navajo taxonomic classification system, the Life Medicines or *azee' tsiin*, "medicine twig(s)". This group contains at least 128 botanical species. There is, however, a core group, the "big medicines", which include *Eriogonum* spp., *Lithospernum* spp., and *Ditaxis cyanophylla*.

Life Medicines are used in the Lifeway sing (one of the Navajo ceremonies) and for treating general injuries such as sprains, strains, fractures, swellings, bruises, wounds, burns, lameness, internal injury, or general body pain. Life Medicines are considered a cure-all and can be administered internally as a cold infusion, a warm infusion, or a dry powder, or externally as a hot or cold poultice or a lotion. Sometimes the roots are chewed. It is best to have six or more of these plants to mix together, though in emergency situations two to four can be used (Mayes VO, Lacy BB. Nanise': A Navajo Herbal. Tsaile, Arizona: Navajo Community College Press; 1989; Wyman LC, Harris SK. Navajo Indian Medical Ethnobotany. University of New Mexico Bulletin, Anthropological Series. 1941;3(5)).

Traditional healing is not the only healing system used by Navajos. The principal investigator for the Navajo Healing Project divides healing in contemporary Navajo society into four distinct systems: Traditional Navajo, Navajo Christian, Navajo Native American Church, and Biomedical (Csordas TJ. The Navajo Healing Project. Med Anthropol Q. 2000;14:463-75). Navajo Christians are of two faiths: Pentecostal Protestant and Roman Catholic. The Pentecostal preacher uses revival meetings and the laying on of hands for healing. The Roman Catholic Church on Navajo reservations combines Navajo and Catholic practices and heals through a prayer group. The Native American Church, which was founded in 1918 in Oklahoma, combines Native and Christian beliefs. The centerpiece of the religion is peyote (*Lophophora williamsii*), a type of cactus considered sacred and the material embodiment of divine power. This plant is considered to have healing properties and enlightens, guides, and teaches the people who partake of it. Meetings take place at night and include prayer, four consumptions of peyote, singing, and visions; Navajo meetings take place in a *hogan* (a traditional lodge).

Navajos, like other contemporary Indians, are not a homogeneous group, and beliefs regarding religion and healing vary. The physician must not assume that, because a person is Navajo, he or she must have particular beliefs, practices, and experiences.

communities are beginning to control their own hospitals, outpatient facilities, and health care programs (2). Generally, any health program proposal brought to a Native community must be formally approved by the tribe before it can be implemented.

The IHS Mission Statement states:

The IHS provides a comprehensive health services delivery system for American Indians and Alaska Natives with opportunity for maximum tribal involvement in developing and managing programs to meet health needs. The goal of IHS is to raise the health status of the American Indian and Alaska Native people to the highest possible level.

To carry out its mission and to attain its goal, IHS: 1) assists Indian tribes in developing their health programs through activities such as health management training, technical assistance and human resource development; 2) facilitates and assists Indian tribes in coordinating health planning, in obtaining and utilizing health resources available through Federal, State and local programs, in operating comprehensive health care services and in health program evaluation; 3) provides comprehensive health care services, including hospital and ambulatory medical care, preventive and rehabilitative services, and development of community sanitation facilities; and 4) serves as the principal Federal advocate for Indians in the health field to ensure comprehensive health services for American Indians and Alaska Native people (2).

IHS is the primary source of medical care for 55% of the Native population. Though most of the people served live on or near reservations, urban care centers provide services to more than 150,000 Indians in 34 cities nationwide. IHS also provides water and waste disposal to 92% of Indian homes; however, 7.5% of Indian homes still lack safe water. Though IHS has constructed health care facilities on many reservations, the average age of these facilities is 32 years, with some older than 60 years. Over one-third of these facilities need replacement to increase clinic space, and many need substantial modernization, particularly those built before the modern emphasis on ambulatory care (2).

Specific Diseases and Mortality

Data collected by the IHS represent approximately 60% of all American Indians and Alaska Natives. These people may or may not use IHS services.

A great deal of racial miscoding of American Indians and Alaska Natives has occurred, forcing IHS to attempt to adjust their data.[4] These factors may result in the underestimation of risk in some categories. In addition, the data track mostly mortality. National and local surveys often do not analyze risk factors and indicators of morbidity and access to care.

The leading causes of death for Indians (i.e., American Indians and Alaska Natives) are diseases of the heart, malignant neoplasms, accidents (motor vehicle and other), diabetes mellitus, chronic liver disease and cirrhosis, cerebrovascular diseases, pneumonia and influenza, suicide, chronic obstructive pulmonary disease, and homicide and legal intervention (Table 4-2).[5] The five leading causes of death for males and for females are listed in Table 4-3.

Striking disparities exist between the health status of American Indians and Alaskan Natives and the general United States population (GUSP). Mortality rates from alcoholism, tuberculosis, diabetes mellitus, accidents,

Table 4-2   Leading Causes of Death (in Descending Order) for American Indians and Alaska Natives and for the General United States Population

American Indians and Alaska Natives	General United States Population
Diseases of the heart	Diseases of the heart
Malignant neoplasms	Malignant neoplasms
Accidents	Cerebrovascular disease
Diabetes mellitus	Chronic obstructive pulmonary disease
Chronic liver disease and cirrhosis	Accidents
Cerebrovascular diseases	Pneumonia and influenza
Pneumonia and influenza	Diabetes mellitus
Suicide	Suicide
Chronic obstructive pulmonary disease	Kidney disease
Homicide and legal intervention	Chronic liver disease and cirrhosis

Data from Indian Health Service 2002 (www.his.gov) and Department of Health and Human Services. Healthy People 2000: Understanding and Improving Health, 2nd ed. Washington, DC: Government Printing Office; 2001.

[4] Health statistics in this section are taken from the IHS publication *Trends in Indian Health, 1998-99* [available on-line from the IHS Web site at www.ihs.gov].

[5] Legal intervention as a cause of death includes, for example, a person killed by a police officer in the line of duty.

Table 4-3   Leading Causes of Death (in Descending Order) for American Indians and Alaska Natives by Gender

Male	Female
Diseases of the heart	Diseases of the heart
Accidents	Malignant neoplasms
Malignant neoplasms	Accidents
Chronic liver disease and cirrhosis	Diabetes mellitus
Suicide	Cerebrovascular diseases

Data from Indian Health Service 2002 (www.his.gov) and Department of Health and Human Services. Healthy People 2000: Understanding and Improving Health, 2nd ed. Washington, DC: Government Printing Office; 2001.

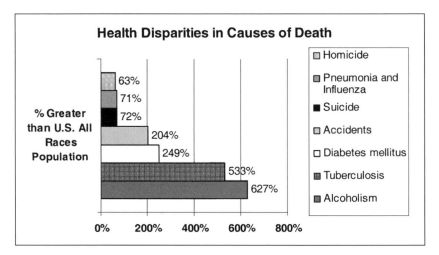

Figure 4-1   Health disparities among American Indians and Alaska Natives compared with the general United States population. (Data from Indian Health Service 2002 [www.his.gov] and Department of Health and Human Services. Healthy People 2010: Understanding and Improving Health, 2nd ed. Washington, DC: Government Printing Office; 2001.)

suicide, pneumonia and influenza, and homicide are significantly higher among Indians (Fig. 4-1).

Alcoholism

Alcoholism is 627% more prevalent in the American Indian and Alaska Native population than in the GUSP. Adjusted data since 1986 give an alcohol-related death ratio for Indians compared with the GUSP of 7:1.

Alcoholism strikes Native men at much higher rates than it does women; for all age groups, males have higher mortality rates from alcoholism than females. Yet mortality rates for females are themselves extremely high. In 1995, overall mortality rates from alcoholism for the female GUSP aged 25 to 74 was <10.0 deaths per 100,000; for female Indians, the rates ranged from 20.6 to 97.8 deaths per 100,000, with the highest rates being for 15 to 24 year olds.

Alcoholism alone can account for many of the differences in overall mortality rates between Native men and women as well as between Natives and non-Natives. Chronic liver disease and cirrhosis, the fifth-leading cause of death for all Natives and the fourth-leading cause of death for males, is due in large part to the high rates of alcoholism. Compared with the GUSP, Indians have almost five times the chance of dying from chronic liver disease and cirrhosis. In addition, for all age groups, Native men have higher rates of chronic liver disease and cirrhosis than Native females. Higher rates of accidents (particularly motor vehicle accidents), suicides, and homicides may also be tied to the high rates of alcoholism in the Native population.

Alcoholism is often called the leading health problem among Indians. Still, a number of misconceptions need to be addressed. First, clarification is necessary as to what is causing alcohol-related mortality and morbidity. It is, in fact, not simply alcoholism but rather a *combination* of alcoholism (alcohol-dependent or chronic drinking behavior, often seen as a dependence on alcohol) and alcohol abuse (sporadic or binge drinking that is not a result of a dependence on alcohol). Alcohol abuse actually causes more sickness and injury than alcoholism itself in both the Native population and the GUSP (23).

A second misconception is that Indians metabolize alcohol differently than other groups. This is belief is common among non-Indians and Indians alike. In one survey of Navajos, for example, 63% of respondents said that Indians have a biological weakness for alcohol (24). No scientific research has substantiated this claim. Instead, studies show that Indians metabolize alcohol as rapidly or more rapidly than other groups and have no phenotypic liver differences (25-27).

That high rates of alcohol-related problems are unique to Indians is a third misconception. Similar rates can be found in other groups that are similar in demographic, geographic, political, and cultural factors (e.g., young, mostly living in rural Western states with delayed access to medical care, lower socio-economic status [SES]) (23).

A fourth misconception is that all Indians drink and they all drink too much. In fact, the prevalence of drinking in the Native population compared with the GUSP is only higher in young men and is actually lower in older men (23). Prevalence of drinking varies among different tribes but is 10% to 30% *lower* than in the GUSP. The major problem seems to reside in a group of individuals who partake in excessive anxiety drinking; their alcoholism rate is two to three times higher than in the GUSP.

The problems surrounding alcoholism and alcohol abuse are not "Indian" at all. Instead, they stem from the same demographic, geographic, and political factors that affect other marginalized peoples. The low SES of Indians is comparable to that of many other ethnic minorities that have problems with alcohol and drug abuse. Many deaths could be prevented if access to care were facilitated in rural Western areas. Finally, the Indian population is generally young, and the young have more drinking problems than any other group. Many non-Indians extrapolate the higher prevalence of drinking among young Indians to the entire Native population, leading to the stereotype that all Indians drink and should be treated as drunks. This stereotype poses the largest problem in treating Indians properly in the medical setting.

Tuberculosis

The mortality rate from tuberculosis for American Indians and Alaska Natives is 533% that for the GUSP. However, the death rate has decreased 82% since 1972, from 10.5 deaths to 1.9 deaths per 100,000 persons. The ratio of Native deaths to white deaths has ranged between 7:1 and 11:1 since 1987.

Pneumonia and Influenza

Aside from tuberculosis, the other infectious diseases that disproportionately affect the Native population are pneumonia and influenza. Deaths from pneumonia and influenza are 71% higher in American Indians and Alaska Natives than in the GUSP. Mortality rates for pneumonia and influenza have decreased in all populations since 1973 but remain 1.7 times higher in the Native population than in the GUSP (22.0 deaths per 100,000 persons versus 12.9 deaths per 100,000 persons). Men aged 65 to 74 and 75 to 84 have slightly higher rates than females.

Diabetes Mellitus

Since 1973, when death data from diabetes began to be collected on a regular basis, the Native population has been shown to have higher rates of diabetes mellitus than the rest of the GUSP. Mortality from the disease is 249% greater for Native people than for the GUSP. For about 20 years, from 1973-93, the mortality rates for diabetes mellitus in Natives ranged from 28.1 to 35.0 deaths per 100,000 persons. After 1993, rates took a sharp incline and for 1994-96 were 46.4 deaths per 100,000 persons. This rate is 3.5 times the diabetes mortality rate for the GUSP, which is 13.3 deaths per 100,000 persons. The ratio of Native deaths due to diabetes mellitus to deaths in the GUSP has varied from 3.0:1 to 3.5:1 since racial miscoding adjustments in 1987. Ratios of diabetes deaths for Natives to whites ranged from 3.3:1 to 4.0:1 during the same period.

Within the Indian population, age-specific diabetes mortality rates for females are higher than for males beginning at age 44, particularly for postmenopausal women. Mortality rates for Native men range from 0.3 to 348.1 deaths per 100,000 males; for women, 3.4 to 491.7 deaths per 100,000 females. Additionally, after age 84, death rates from diabetes for men drop, whereas for women they continue at a high rate, even increasing slightly. These trends differ from those for the GUSP, where female mortality rates stay consistently below the male rates. Clearly, Native women have a heightened risk of death due to this disease compared with other women or Native men. Diabetes mellitus is the fourth-leading cause of death for Native women, yet is not in the top five for men.

Arguments have been made that Indians have a genetic predisposition to this disorder, particularly non-insulin-dependent diabetes mellitus (NIDDM), the diabetes type that normally begins in adulthood. Neel (28) was the first to argue that a "thrifty genotype" is responsible for the high rates. He argued that genetic adaptations for storing energy in times of famine while leading a feast-or-famine lifestyle would predispose people to diabetes who are living a more modern lifestyle. Weiss and co-workers (29) built on this theory, saying that the "thrifty gene" represents an altered form of lipid metabolism, based on the fact that cardiovascular disease, hypertension, and stroke were not found in greater proportions in the Native population, whereas NIDDM, obesity, gallstones, gallbladder cancer, and abnormalities of cholesterol metabolism were. Another possibility for this genotype is that it is "glucose-sparing" because surviving the Bering Strait migration would have required a diet high in protein, moderate in fat, and very low in glucose (30).

Ritenbaugh and Goodby (31) compared modern lifestyles with those of hunters and agriculturalists during traditional times. The hunting lifestyle included a diet based on animal sources that were low in carbohydrates, low in dietary fiber, moderate in fat, and high in protein. There were high energy demands for activity and warmth. An agricultural lifestyle included a diet high in carbohydrates and dietary fiber, moderate in protein, and low in fat. High energy demands were necessary for work. In both of these lifestyles there would have been seasonal macronutrient shortages. The modern lifestyle generally includes a diet of store-bought groceries that is high in carbohydrates, moderate in fat and protein, and low in dietary fiber. There are low energy demands for work and sedentary leisure time activities such as watching television. There are no seasonal macronutrient shortages.

The "thrifty gene" hypothesized to account for the overwhelming prevalence of diabetes among Indians has not been found. Lifestyle changes, however, are obvious and tied directly to life on a reservation, complete with commodity food (government-provided cheese, canned foods, and powdered milk, for example, given as part of social welfare programs) and forced assimilation to Euro-American culture. Today's lifestyles, particularly those of people in the lower socioeconomic classes, do not only allow for obesity but encourage it. Changes in exercise habits are the most successful way of decreasing the prevalence of diabetes in adult populations (32). Interventions for preventing and treating diabetes in this population must focus on lifestyle changes.

Diseases of the Heart, Cerebrovascular Disease, and Chronic Obstructive Pulmonary Disease

American Indian and Alaska Native mortality rates for diseases of the heart, cerebrovascular disease, and chronic obstructive pulmonary disease, while lower than those for the GUSP, are increasing and approaching the GUSP rates.

Cancer

Mortality rates for cancer are also increasing among the Native population. Malignant neoplasm or cancer deaths were once much lower in the American Indian and Alaska Native population than in the rest of the GUSP. In fact, in 1977-79, rates of cancer death in the Native population were as low as 80.2 deaths per 100,000 persons compared with the GUSP rate of 133.8 deaths per 100,000 persons. Rates for the Native population have increased since 1977-79 to 116.6 deaths per 100,000 persons. Native men have higher death rates from cancer than women after age 55, though women's rates are higher in the two decades before. The leading sites for cancer deaths in Native males are trachea, lung, and bronchus, then prostate, colon, stomach, and liver; for females, trachea, lung, and bronchus, then breast, colon, ovary, and pancreas. For all men in the United States, the leading causes of cancer deaths are lung and bronchus, prostate, colon and rectum, pancreas, and non-Hodgkin's lymphoma; for all women, lung and bronchus, breast, colon and rectum, pancreas, and ovary (33).[6]

An important difference between the American Indian and Alaska Native population and the rest of the United States population is the percentage of people with cancer who die from the disease. When cancer incidence and mortality rates are compared across racial/ethnic groups, this disparity becomes apparent. In the white population, overall 41% of cancer patients die from the disease, 43% of men and 39% of women. In the black population, 49% of cancer patients die from the disease, 50% of men and 49% of women. In the American Indian and Alaska Native population, 52% of cancer patients die from the disease, 55% of men and 49% of women. Asian/Pacific Islander and Hispanic populations both have lower rates than the white population (34). It is very possible that these higher Native death rates, particularly for Native men, are due to barriers to access to care, later stage at diagnosis, and quality of care.

Accidents

Mortality rates from accidents are 204% greater in the American Indian and Alaska Native population compared with the GUSP. Deaths from accidents have decreased by over 50% since 1972; the decrease has slowed over the last ten years. The 1994-96 Native accident rate of 92.6 deaths per 100,000 persons is more than triple the GUSP rate of 30.5 deaths per 100,000 persons. The mortality rate for Indians for motor vehicle accidents is 54.0 deaths per 100,000 persons, which represents 58.3% of all accidental deaths; the motor vehicle accident mortality rate for the GUSP is 16.3 deaths per 100,000

---

[6] Because the leading causes of cancer death for Indians and all races are taken from different sources, there are slightly different groupings of cancer. Trachea, lung, and bronchus in Indians are part of one grouping, while lung and bronchus in all races is the same grouping. Also, colon cancer is listed singly in Indians but is grouped with rectal cancer in all races. Because trachea and rectal cancers account for far less cancer death than the other cancers within the groupings, these groupings can be considered analogous.

persons, which represents 53.4% of all accidental deaths. Death rates from accidents are higher for Native men than for Native women.

Suicide

Mortality rates from suicide are 72% higher for the American Indian and Alaska Native population compared with the GUSP. Rates have fluctuated over time; the 19.3 deaths per 100,000 persons in 1994-96 was an increase of 21% compared with the rates for 1984-86. Within the Native population, suicides account for more male than female deaths. Male death rates are highest for 25 to 34 year olds (66.7 deaths per 100,000 persons) and for 15 to 24 year olds (53.5 deaths per 100,000 persons).

Homicide

Deaths from homicides are 63% higher among the American Indian and Alaska Native population than for the GUSP. Homicide rates have decreased 37% since 1973, to 15.3 deaths per 100,000 persons. This rate is still 1.6 times higher than the GUSP rate of 9.4 deaths per 100,000 persons and 2.8 times higher than the white rate of 5.5 deaths per 100,000 persons. Homicide rates for Native males are much higher than for Native females. Native males aged 15 to 24 and 25 to 34 have exceptionally high rates of homicide deaths (both 40.0 deaths per 100,000 men) as do men aged 35 to 44 (36.5 deaths per 100,000 men). Homicide rates for Native females are highest for women aged 35 to 44 (10.8 deaths per 100,000 females) and for women aged 25 to 34 (10.1 deaths per 100,000 females). Firearm death rates parallel homicide rates, probably not coincidentally.

Infant Mortality

Though not a leading cause of death in the American Indian and Alaska Native population as a whole, there is a disparity in infant mortality between the Native population and the GUSP. Infant mortality has decreased 58% since 1973, from 22.2 deaths per 1000 live births to 9.3 deaths per 1000 live births in 1994-96. This rate is 22% higher than the rate of 7.6 deaths per 1000 live births for the GUSP and is 1.5 times that for whites. The rates for sudden infant death syndrome (SIDS) in Native populations are 2.2 times higher than the rate for the GUSP and 2.9 times higher than the rate for whites.

Health Disparities Today

It is clear that some of the disparities in health between the American Indian and Alaska Native population and the general United States population have decreased in the past 25 years. However, as has been seen in the foregoing discussion of various diseases and causes of death, disparities still exist. Some mortality outcomes, particularly for alcoholism and diabetes, are increasing in the Native population, and disparities in health are in some cases becoming greater. These outcomes must be addressed vigorously and reversed.

Language and Communication

When treating the American Indian or Alaska Native patient, it is necessary to understand some of the cultural barriers to effective communication and, therefore, treatment and compliance. Communication must be seen as both verbal and nonverbal. The most obvious problem that may exist in verbal communication is a language barrier. Many people believe that all Natives in the United States speak English or that their traditional languages are "dead". In fact, there are many monolingual speakers of Native languages, particularly in the older generation. There are also bilingual speakers of Native languages whose second language is not English but Spanish, French, or Russian, depending on the area of the country. If interpreters are needed, it may be difficult to find trained medical professionals, and family or community members may have to be used.

A possible problem between Natives and non-Native medical practitioners is the pace or speed of conversation. Many Indians consider speaking too quickly a sign of disrespect. Words themselves are sacred and should not be wasted. Because of this, pauses are very common between speakers and interruptions are considered rude. When speaking with a Native patient, a physician should pause before replying to ensure that the patient has finished speaking, decide carefully what needs to be said, then speak in a measured deliberate manner.

Another sign of disrespect is speaking too loudly. Within the United States, there are regional differences in pace and loudness of conversation. For example, people in the Northeast tend to speak more quickly and loudly than people in the West. Tone of conversations can also be different.

Sarcasm, for example, is reserved for certain relations, such as in-laws, and is not generally considered funny. Sarcastic remarks are considered rude, particularly when talking about traditional beliefs.

A final verbal communication issue is taboos against using specific words or discussing particular topics. A common Native taboo prohibits speaking the name of a deceased individual. It is believed that speaking the name calls the person's spirit, which can bring misfortune and harm. Taking a family medical history can therefore be difficult. One way to avoid the taboo is to use kinship terminology, such as "maternal grandmother". Another common taboo is against speaking too much about an illness, which is believed to make that illness worse. Though there are some common taboos, many more are specific to particular groups. For example, among the Navajo, the terms "please" and "thank you" are not commonly used. "Please" is considered a sign of begging and is not necessary. "Thank you" is an unnecessary term because of social obligations.

Communication can also be nonverbal. Prolonged intense eye contact in many Native groups is considered rude. In mainstream United States culture, eye contact while someone is speaking is considered polite and correct. This same eye contact is inappropriate to many Indians. This is not to say that a person should deliberately look away when talking to an Indian patient, but rather that staring while talking is not the best course of action.

Gender Roles and Reproductive Health

Many issues surround Native male-female communication. Certain topics should not be discussed between the sexes, particularly issues surrounding reproductive health. Birth itself is often considered a part of the female domain and should not involve men, including male doctors. Even seeing a woman without her clothes can be considered wrong for any man. This became an issue for one of the authors when helping to evaluate breast and cervical cancer education materials. These materials could not include pictures of women without clothing, particularly on the cover.

Menstruation is a unique part of the female domain, particularly so among some Indian nations such as the Lakota. Traditionally, during menstruation women were secluded from men in the *isnati* (menstruation hut). During this time, women were not permitted to cook or touch food, to come near men or weapons, or to deal with any ritual paraphernalia or herbal medicines. The touch of menstruating woman was thought to render those objects useless. Though menstrual taboos may not be as strict today, restrictions remain (14). For example, menstruating women are not permitted to attend certain ceremonies, including *Yuwipi* ceremonies and sun dances, and may not be welcome in certain homes. If a menstruating woman is ill, it may be difficult to treat her, particularly if the physician is male or if objects considered ritualistic are kept at the clinic or hospital. It may be necessary, particularly with traditional women, to ensure that a female physician is available or, at a minimum, that another woman is present during examination and discussion.

Family Structure

Though it is not usual in mainstream United States culture for family members to be present during medical consultations, it is common in many Indian cultures. Family members who are not permitted to be a part of a medical consultation feel that they are being disrespected. Patients may be uncooperative and not totally forthcoming if their family members are not permitted to be with them, especially if there are gender differences between the patient and physician. Health is not simply an individual issue; rather, it is something of which the entire family is a part. Family members should never be shut out at the sole discretion of the physician; the patient must be consulted in this matter. For example, in certain remote areas of reservations in the Southwest, it is necessary to airlift patients with certain conditions to major cities, such as Phoenix or Tucson, particularly when surgery is required. Transportation for family members is not often provided and may become an important issue for the patient and the family (Case 4-1).

Another family issue that can become a barrier to effective treatment deals with taking a medical history. Besides the taboo of not mentioning the name of a deceased individual (discussed above), Native views of lineage may present obstacles. Within mainstream United States culture, most people trace their heritage through both the mother's and father's side of the family. This is known as bilateral descent. Many Native people, on the other hand, trace their lineage through the mother's (matrilineal) or father's (patrilineal) side, but not both. People who are on one particular side of the

---

CASE 4-1   A 72-YEAR-OLD AMERICAN INDIAN MALE WHO NEEDS SURGERY AND IS SEPARATED FROM HIS FAMILY

Will Firestone, a 72-year-old Indian male who lives on a reservation in Central Arizona, is taken by medical helicopter to a major hospital, approximately 4 hr away by car, for emergency double-bypass surgery. Because of IHS rules, no family member is permitted to accompany him. His family does not own a car and cannot afford bus fare to the hospital or lodging nearby.

Mr Firestone was hospitalized for several weeks. His English was poor and he could not adequately explain his complaints; no interpreter was available. He believed that family members could have told medical personnel what was needed to help him. Because he felt that his concerns were not being heard, he felt no need to comply with the instructions that doctors were giving him. Once he returned home, he did not make the suggested behavioral changes to help his heart condition. He said that his traditional diet and lifestyle were the best things for him, and that if doctors knew more about them they would approve of his course of action.

DISCUSSION

This unfortunate situation could have been remedied by allowing a family member, preferably one who speaks better English, to accompany the patient on the airlift to the hospital, with explanations provided to the IHS later. Arrangements for the family member to stay at the hospital could also have been made. In this way, Mr Firestone's views and concerns could have been communicated fully to his physicians, and together the patient and doctors could have agreed on the best course of treatment.

---

family are considered a part of the lineage and people on the other side are not. Therefore if a patient is asked if a certain disease is present within his or her family and the disease is present on the side of the family not considered a part of the lineage, then that history of the disease would not be mentioned. To avoid confusion, it is necessary to specifically ask if anyone on the patient's mother's side or father's side (or mother's relatives or father's relatives) has had the disease.

Developing Effective Patient-Physician Relationships and Treatment Plans

If effective communication is established during the patient-physician encounter, it becomes possible for both parties to explain what they believe is the best course of action. Each party has his or her own beliefs about what the disease is, how it was caused, and how it should be treated. Both parties can share their ideas of effective treatment regimens, though these ideas may be very different and based on different kinds of medical and cultural systems (e.g., naturalistic versus personalistic). This sharing is imperative, especially when the ideas are in conflict (see Chapter 1 for further discussion about exploring a patient's explanatory model of illness).

Many Native peoples believe that there are two different types of disease, Indian and white, with some overlap between the two. Indian diseases are those that have always affected Native peoples of the Americas and are treated most effectively through traditional medicine. White diseases are those that have been brought to the Americas by whites and are treated most effectively through biomedicine. An overlap between these two categories comprises diseases that have been treated with some efficacy by both traditional medicine and biomedicine. Cancer, for example, has been treated effectively through biomedicine but has also been treated effectively through traditional medicine, particularly in later stages and for some of the nonphysical symptoms (Box 4-2).

Some people combine treatment modalities, wishing to use the most efficacious treatments of each medical system. Physicians must be open to the idea of combining medical treatments or simply using treatments from another medical system. It is important that the physician know if a patient is planning to use traditional medicine of any kind, particularly herbal remedies that may interact with drug regimens. Physicians must ask about the use of traditional medicine and not discount its efficacy. Many Native patients will use traditional medicine regardless of their physician's recommendations, so it is necessary for the physician to ask about them and work treatment plans around them. By being open to other medical systems, physicians will be better able to treat their Native patients, and compliance may go up if the patients see this open relationship.

Box 4-2   Native Beliefs about Cancer

Csordas examined Navajo beliefs related to cancer and discovered that it is not seen as a group of discrete entities (e.g., breast cancer, lung cancer) but rather as one large disease that can affect the body in different places (Csordas TJ. The sore that does not heal: cause and concept in the Navajo experience of cancer. J Anthropological Research. 1989;45:457-85). Navajos place the origins of cancer in the second world of creation (the Yellow World), where it is the result of sexual transgressions such as incest, homosexuality, and trans-sexuality, and thereby linked to sexually transmitted diseases. Another possible cause in the Yellow World is the attempt to control nature and the misuse of natural powers. This links cancer most specifically to lightning, but also to radiation and dangerous chemicals. Navajos, asked about their cancer, reported several causes, not just one. The terms used to describe cancer can be translated as "the sore that does not heal" and "keeps on rotting".

McPheron-Alex studied the beliefs of the Pasqua Yaqui about cancer, especially lung cancer (McPheron-Alex T. Predisposing Cultural Factors among American Indian Populations Related to Cancer Occurrence. Master's thesis. Tucson: University of Arizona; 1996). The Yaqui belief system allows that cancer can be caused by taboo violation and/or supernatural causes. This belief is flexible enough to allow for unhealthy nutrition and cigarette smoking as causal agents. Past transgressions or witchcraft can also cause cancer. The subject is generally avoided in conversation because talking about cancer may cause one to get it—in other words, give cancer "power and recognition" (McPheron-Alex, *op. cit.*).

Makosky studied the attitudes of female Indian college students towards cancer (Makosky CA. Perspectives on the Causes of Breast Cancer among American Indian Women College Students. Unpublished Master's thesis. Tempe: Arizona State University; 1998). Cancer was viewed as a "white disease" brought to Indians by Europeans. The students' understanding of cancer was biomedical in nature (i.e., participants equated "white diseases" with biomedicine), although their beliefs did not directly correspond with biomedical cancer models. Participants noted various causes of cancer, including heredity, diet, exposure to harmful things in the environment (e.g., radiation), lifestyle choices (e.g., smoking), not taking care of oneself, birth control pills, power lines, chemicals in foods, sugar, UV rays, and x-rays. Many of the young women, however; said they had no idea what caused cancer or

---

Box 4-2 (continued)

why. Most felt that cancer is always fatal. Some, in particular, felt that cancer would be fatal for them because they are Indian and cannot get the best health care.

Regarding cancer treatment, the students believed that biomedicine and traditional medicine could both be used. In fact, a combination of these two healing approaches would produce the best outcomes, even if that outcome were only longer life, not an escape from death. They also noted that physical symptoms would be best treated by biomedicine, whereas emotional and spiritual healing needed to be addressed through traditional medicine. Less than half of the students said they would go to one type of healer exclusively.

It is clear that more information is needed on Native beliefs surrounding cancer (and other illnesses) before it is possible to develop the most efficacious treatments for this group.

Conclusion

For most Indians, medicine and religion are tightly interwoven. Many Indians believe that illness has its cause rooted in the spirit world, and that the spirit world must likewise be involved in its cure. For these reasons, and because of a deep-seated distrust of many Western practices, including biomedicine, many conventional treatments may not be acceptable to Native patients. Still, if biomedical concepts can be explained in terms more in keeping with Native beliefs, it may be possible to bridge the gap.

Although this chapter has discussed general beliefs and practices of Native groups, it is important to realize that each individual Indian nation has its own distinct practices and beliefs. There are many resources available to those who plan to work with Native peoples. Aside from the vast published literature, many Indian communities have cultural and health advisory boards that can provide detailed and contemporary information. In addition, many Indian communities have museums and cultural centers that can provide general information on historical and contemporary issues. The bottom line is: Ask Questions. The information you or your patients need *is* available; it is just a matter of knowing where to look.

Summary of Special Issues in Care of American Indians and Alaska Natives

Verbal and Nonverbal Communications

- Verbal communication
  - Some older Native people may not speak English
    - Trained interpreters are an important resource
  - Speaking too quickly is a sign of disrespect
    - Pauses are common and should not be interrupted
    - Pausing before answering is a sign of respect and thoughtfulness
  - Speaking too loudly is a sign of disrespect
  - Taboos exist against using certain words or discussing certain topics
    - Taboos vary among different Indian nations
      - Ask questions of someone who is familiar and understands the culture
      - Common taboos to avoid
        - Using the name of a deceased person
        - Speaking too much about a specific illness
        - Certain topics, such as reproductive health, are not discussed between genders
      - Prolonged intense eye contact is rude

Family Members, Lineage, Models, and Treatment

- It is common to have family members present at medical consultation.
- Many traditional Native people trace their lineage primarily through the mother or father, but not both.
  - A physician may have to ask specifically about family history from the "other" side.
- Both the patient and physician should offer his or her explanatory model of illness (or health).
- Providers should be open to combining treatment modalities (biomedical and traditional).

Views on Science and Medicine

- Mistrust of biomedicine arises, in part, from historic persecution of Native people.
- Native people have views about their origins that are distinctly different from evolutionary theories.
- Religion and medicine are intimately intertwined, thus resulting in a personalistic system of health and wellness (as compared with naturalistic system of biomedicine).
  - This view assumes multiple levels of causality.
  - Illness is most often beyond the control of the patient.
  - Positive actions can be used as prevention.
- Illness is seen as misfortune.
- If biomedicine can be explained using more personalistic terms, it is possible to bridge the gap between personalistic and naturalistic systems.

Summary of Obstacles to Health Care Delivery in American Indian and Alaska Native Patients

- Low socioeconomic status, may not have private health insurance
- Residence in isolated rural area, thus increasing rates of mortality from otherwise treatable accidents and illnesses
- Illiteracy issues and language barriers (particularly among the elderly)
- Mistrust of Western medicine due to long-standing differences with the United States government
- Communication differences
- Native explanatory models of health and illness may not be understood by treating physician

REFERENCES

1. Berkhofer RF Jr. The White Man's Indian: Images of the American Indian from Columbus to Present. New York: Knopf; 1978.
2. Indian Health Service Web site (www.ihs.gov).
3. Mihesuah DA. American Indian identities: issues of individual choice and development. In: Champagne D, ed. Contemporary Native American Cultural Issues. Walnut Creek, California: AltaMira Press; 1999:13-38.
4. Utter J. American Indians: Answers to Today's Questions. Lake Ann, Michigan: National Woodlands Publishing; 1993.
5. Crawford DH. The Invisible Enemy: A Natural History of Viruses. Oxford: OUP; 2000.
6. Watts S. Epidemics and History: Disease, Power and Imperialism. New Haven: Yale University Press; 1997.
7. Prucha FP, ed. Documents of United States Indian Policy, 2nd ed (expanded). Lincoln: University of Nebraska Press; 1990.
8. Josephy AM. Jr. Now That the Buffalo's Gone: A Study of Today's American Indians. Norman: University of Oklahoma Press; 1984.
9. Nabokov P. Native American Testimony: A Chronicle of Indian-White Relations from Prophesy to the Present: 1492-2000. New York: Penguin Books; 2000.
10. Deloria V Jr. Red Earth, White Lies: Native Americans and the Myth of Scientific Fact. New York: Scribner's; 1996.
11. Powers WK. War Dance: Plains Indian Musical Performance. Tucson: University of Arizona Press; 1990.
12. Oswalt WH. This Land was Theirs: A Study of Native Americans, 7th ed. Boston: McGraw- Hill/Mayfield; 2002.
13. Foster GM. Disease etiologies in non-Western medical systems. In: Brown, PJ, ed. Understanding and Applying Medical Anthropology. Mountain View: Mayfield; 1998:110-7.
14. Powers M. Oglala Women: Myth, Ritual, and Reality. Chicago: University of Chicago Press; 1986.
15. Powers WK. Oglala Religion. Lincoln: University of Nebraska Press; 1975.
16. Basso KH. The Cibecue Apache. Prospect Heights: Waveland Press; 1970.

17. Goodwin G. Myths and Tales of the White Mountain Apache. Tucson: University of Arizona Press; 1994.

18. Bierhorst J, ed. The Sacred Path: Spells, Prayers and Power Songs of the American Indians. New York: Quill; 1983.

19. Garbarino MS, Sasso RF. Native American Heritage, 3rd ed. Prospect Heights: Waveland Press; 1994.

20. Reichard GA. Navaho Religion: A Study of Symbolism. New York: Bollingen Foundation; 1950.

21. Momaday NS. The Way to Rainy Mountain. Albuquerque: University of New Mexico Press; 1969.

22. Johnson G. Indian Tribes' Creationists Thwart Archaeologists. www.santafe.edu/~johnson/articles.creation.html; 22 October 1996.

23. May PA. The epidemiology of alcohol abuse among American Indians: the mythical and real properties. In: Champagne D, ed. Contemporary Native American Cultural Issues. Walnut Creek, California: AltaMira Press; 1999:227-44.

24. May PA, Smith MB. Some Navajo Indian opinions about alcohol abuse and prohibition: a survey and recommendations for policy. J Stud Alcohol. 1987;49:324-34.

25. Bennion LJ, Li TK. Alcohol metabolism in American Indians and whites: lack of racial differences in metabolic state and liver alcohol dehydrogenase. N Engl J Med. 1976; 284:9-13.

26. Leiber CS. Metabolism of ethanol and alcoholism: racial and acquired factors. Ann Intern Med. 1972;76:326-7.

27. Reed TE, Kalant H, Gibbins RJ, et al. Alcohol and acetaldehyde metabolism in Caucasians, Chinese, and Amerinds. Can Med Assoc J. 1976;115:851-8.

28. Neel JV. Diabetes mellitus: a "thrifty" genotype rendered detrimental by "progress." Am J Hum Genet. 1962;14:353-62.

29. Weiss KM, Ferrell RE, Hanis CL. A New World syndrome of metabolic diseases with a genetic and evolutionary basis. Yearbook of Physical Anthropology. 1984;27:153-78.

30. Schaefer O, Crockford PM, Romanowski B. Normalization effect of preceding protein meals on "diabetic" oral glucose tolerance in Eskimos. Can Med Assoc J. 1972;107:733-8.

31. Ritenbaugh C, Goodby C-S. Beyond the thrifty gene: metabolic implications of prehistoric migration into the New World. In: Brown PJ, ed. Understanding and Applying Medical Anthropology. Mountain View, California: Mayfield.1998:46-52.

32. Diabetes Prevention Program Research Group. Reduction in the incidence of type 2 diabetes with lifestyle intervention or Metformin. N Engl J Med. 2002;346:393-403.

33. American Cancer Society. Cancer Facts and Figures, 2001. Atlanta: American Cancer Society; 2001.

34. Mitka M. Disparity in cancer statistics changing. JAMA. 2002;287:703-4.

5

Care of Asian Americans

JEAN LAU CHIN, EdD

JUDYANN BIGBY, MD

The specific health care needs of Asian Americans and Pacific Islanders are often overlooked because their numbers are small and they are viewed as a model minority. Too often Americans of Asian and Pacific Islander descent have been classified as "other", thus rendering them, for practical purposes, invisible. This practice has obscured our understanding of the health care challenges facing these populations, of the within-group diversity, and of the sociocultural factors that influence health and wellness. Some of the populations that have been lumped into the group "Asian/Pacific Islander" are indigenous to the United States and have had to fight for recognition as native people. Other populations have a long history in America and represent second- and third-generation Americans from many Asian countries. Many others face specific challenges because of their adjustment to immigration. In this chapter we discuss the health care of Asian Americans—those who are descendents of, or immigrants from, countries that are considered part of Asia.

The values, beliefs, identity, and behaviors of any ethnic group are evolutionary and developmental. Vast differences exist among individuals and ethnic groups in the practice of, and adherence to, their cultural beliefs and practices despite a broad embracing of cultural principles. Although second- and third-generation Asian Americans are less likely than first-generation immigrants to be familiar with traditional Asian health beliefs or to practice Asian health behaviors, many of these beliefs and practices are sustained across the generations at a less conscious and overt level. For white immigrants to the United States, acculturation and blending into mainstream society have usually been of prime importance; however, biculturalism and retention of culture from one's country of origin is more often valued by Asian Americans and other communities of color.

Demographics

According to the Census Bureau, Asian Americans comprised 4.2% of the total United States population in 2000, numbering nearly 12 million.* It is projected that Asian Americans will comprise more than 10% of the population by 2050. Yet, this unitary figure is inadequate to capture the diversity within the Asian American population that has its origin in more than 50 countries and ethnic groups.

The majority of Asian Americans are concentrated in fewer than ten states including California, Washington, Hawaii, New York, New Jersey, Illinois, and Texas. The largest ethnic groups include Chinese Americans, Filipino Americans, Asian Indian Americans, Vietnamese Americans, and Korean Americans (1). More than 50% of Asian Americans are foreign born. Lumping ethnic groups into one category can obscure opposing trends and lead to incorrect conclusions about disease states and trends (2). Many resources document the heterogeneity of Asian Americans and their population demographics (3,4). Native Hawaiians and Pacific Islanders are officially classified as a group indigenous to the United States and are only mentioned in passing in this chapter.

Historical Perspective

Asians have immigrated to the United States to improve economic conditions, to escape from political oppression and war, and/or to attain higher education. The United States has received immigrants to meet economic needs for cheap labor or to offer political support for the democratic societies. The sociopolitical contexts of Asian American groups have differed depending on the major period of immigration during which they came to the United States. An understanding of the bilateral interaction of these forces on the adjustment, views, and acculturation of different Asian American groups is essential to cross-cultural care because of their influence on access, utilization, and adherence to medical therapies. At the same time, vast within-group differences and heterogeneity exist.

Racism and the differential treatment of peoples of color in the United States are interwoven with the political and social rationale for welcoming

---

* Population statistics throughout this chapter are from the 2000 census.

immigrants to this country. A comparison of the long-standing "melting pot" view of America with the more recent concept of America as a "tossed salad" brings out two contrasting views about how immigrants ought to adjust to their experience. The "melting pot" concept, long applicable to white immigrants, suggests and embraces the notion of eliminating cultural uniqueness and difference as immigrants from a variety of countries and cultures "melt together" to become Americans. The "tossed salad" view, on the other hand, embraces the notion of cultural difference in enriching the lives of all Americans as people from diverse backgrounds mix and blend together but never lose their distinct, unique qualities. For nonwhite immigrants, this is crucial to the social realities of their experience.

Unfortunately, United States legislation, dating as far back as the 1800s, reflects social policy that discriminates against racial and ethnic immigrant groups who are nonwhite. In particular, legislation has codified immigration policies that have been discriminatory toward Chinese and other Asian groups, resulting in quotas, closer scrutiny, and extra hurdles for citizenship unparalleled for any other racial or ethnic group. Policies have favored different Asian groups depending on the political leanings of their countries of origin. Easing of quotas has consistently shown an ebb and flow with labor shortages and times of economic recession, contributing to feelings of exploitation and mistrust.

Many Western religious groups (e.g., Christian missionaries) have attempted to impose their beliefs and practices onto Asian cultures in the misbelief that they were improving and enriching the culture. Missionaries have often viewed Christianity as the salvation for the unbelieving and the superstitious masses of Asians despite the presence of Buddhism, Taoism, Hinduism, and Shinto within the Asian cultures. Western media and culture have been transplanted to Asia. Western customs viewed as "modernizing" have been brought forward as necessary to move Asians away from "old-fashioned" beliefs and cultures, often viewed as backward and outdated.

Like other nonwhite groups in the United States, Asian Americans have been subjected to racism and derogatory stereotypes. Asians have often been portrayed as immoral and inferior to those in the West, if not subhuman (e.g., images portraying Asian women as prostitutes, rumors of Chinese restaurants serving dog and cat meat), creating perceptions of Asians as primitive, heathen, and hedonistic. The net effect has had significant and often adverse impact on the psyche of Asian Americans in their identity development and their adjustment to American culture. In the opinion of some, these negative stereotypes made it easier for the United States during World War II to justify the internment of Japanese American citizens and the dropping of the atomic bomb on Hiroshima. Later, the Korean and Vietnam Wars provided Americans with images of Asians as "gooks" that were reinforced in popular motion pictures. These experiences have reinforced Asian group solidarity while also resulting in some hostility toward Westerners.

Nothing can capture the full extent of the vast differences and opposing world-views and values of Eastern and Western cultures. These differences form the basis for mutual misunderstanding and mistrust. Asian values that promote group solidarity, modesty, and deference to authority have sometimes been exploited by Westerners who take Asian adherence to this philosophy as indicators of passivity and weakness. The retreat by Asian Americans to in-group isolation, fueled as much by a racist society as by a need to retain cultural values and beliefs, has in turn furthered the perception of Asians as mistrustful and exotic.

Immigration Patterns

Chinese Americans

The immigration of Chinese and Filipino sailors as galley slaves to the Caribbean and Latin America dates back to the 1760s. Chinese, Japanese, Koreans, Filipinos, and Asian Indians (the "coolie" trade) migrated in greater numbers to the British colonies after Parliament abolished slavery in 1833. An increase in Asian immigration to the United States began during the 1850s in response to the California Gold Rush.

In the 1860s, the decision to build the Transcontinental Railroad coincided with floods in the Guangdong and Fujian provinces and fueled the massive immigration of Cantonese Chinese to the United States in response to the recruitment of cheap labor. Famine, pestilence, and political turmoil also propelled vast numbers of Chinese to the United States as temporary "sojourners" intending to make their fortunes and return home. In California at that time Chinese immigrants made up 75% of the farm worker population. Chinese were perceived to be competing with whites for work and, as a result, white workers pushed for the exclusion of Chinese laborers. The Chinese Exclusion Act of 1882 suspended the entry of

Chinese laborers into the United States. Because other groups were not completely barred, the Chinese have the dubious distinction of being the first ethnic group to be barred legally from immigrating to the United States. The Act also denied Chinese the opportunity to become naturalized citizens.

The Chinese Exclusion Act was repealed in 1943, but under the National Origins Quota Act immigration was limited. Chinese Americans were not permitted in many occupations, including gold mining, and deprived of many legal rights, giving rise to the fear of persecution and the popular saying "You don't have a Chinaman's chance". Consequently, early Chinese immigrants resorted to opening laundries and restaurants as the only means for social and economic survival. Educational attainment became the means through which advancement was possible and coincided with the Asian value of education.

It was not until 1965 with the Family Reunification Act that Chinese Americans were allowed to reunite with family members, many of whom had migrated to Hong Kong from China. Later waves of Chinese immigrants came from Taiwan, primarily to pursue higher education.

The Chinese have immigrated from many countries including the People's Republic of China, Hong Kong, Taiwan, Thailand, Indonesia, Vietnam, and Singapore. These groups have different sociopolitical histories and immigration experiences, all of which affect health care utilization. The Chinese are the largest Asian ethnic group (2.7 million) in the United States.

Japanese Americans

Japanese Americans number approximately 1 million. Japanese immigration began as early as the 1850s. Many became gardeners because of restriction on participation in other fields and for economic survival. The National Origins Act barred Japanese and other Asians from entering the United States after 1924. The internment experience of World War II devastated the psychological fabric of the communities. Believing they had been accepted as full citizens, most Japanese Americans were horrified to find their civil rights violated and eliminated. No white American group was stripped of possessions and rights even though the United States was at war not only with Japan but with Germany and Italy. It seemed clear that race was the differential factor in the treatment of Japanese Americans.

Filipino Americans

Filipino Americans make up the second-largest Asian American ethnic group (2.3 million). Filipino immigration began between 1903 and 1910 and was characterized by three waves. Because of the occupation of the Philippines during the Spanish-American War, Filipinos were considered American nationals and many made their way to the United States. Shortly after World War I, many Filipinos came to the mainland as laborers, replacing the niche left by Chinese and Japanese immigrants. The third wave began after 1965 when the quota system was discontinued.

Southeast Asians

Beginning in 1975 with the fall of Saigon and the end of the Vietnam War, Southeast Asian migration increased dramatically. Vietnamese refugees constituted the largest of these refugees, initially to escape war, political persecution, and famine. Cambodians and Laotians made up about 20% of refugees. A second wave came between 1978 and 1980, as political turmoil escalated in Cambodia, Vietnam, and Laos. The Hmong, displaced from their rural locations in Southeast Asia, spent time in refugee camps in Thailand before arriving in the United States. The experiences of these refugees may color their perceptions about American health care (see, for example, Anne Fadiman's *The Spirit Catches You and You Fall Down* and the Hmong's fears of American doctors based on a refugee camp rumor that American doctors eat human brains). Refugees escaping in small, overcrowded boats, often subject to torture or rape, characterized the migration of Southeast Asians, as well as their detainment in camps before resettlement to the United States. Trauma coupled with poverty and illiteracy made the adjustment of Southeast Asian immigrants difficult.

There are 1.2 million Vietnamese in the United States, and approximately 200,000 each of Cambodians, Laotians, and Hmong.

Asian Indians

Asian Indians have immigrated to North America since the 1800s when states such as Massachusetts developed a healthy trade with India. During the British Raj, famine and poor economic conditions pushed many young men to immigrate to the United States to find work to support their families back home. Subsequently, Asian Indians came as both laborers and students. This immigration was challenged in federal court over the question of their racial classification (fueled by United States support of the occupation of India by Great Britain). The right of Asian Indians to become naturalized citizens was also challenged due to their nonwhite status, but this was allowed in 1946. During the 1980s and 1990s the United States saw its largest wave of Asian Indian immigration, consisting primarily of the well-educated and professionals. There are 1.9 million Asian Indians in the United States.

Other Asian Groups

Other Asian groups who have immigrated to the United States in significant numbers include Koreans, Thais, and South Asians other than Indians (Malaysians, Sri Lankans, Pakistanis, and Bangladeshis).

Impact of Bias and Sociopolitical Experience

By Asians Toward Westerners

Colonization of the countries in the East by Western powers and racism in the United States did much to influence the sense of mistrust and feelings of domination and oppression by Asian Americans toward Westerners. Traumatic histories because of sociopolitical factors (e.g., war, internment camps, torture, famine) prior to migration have been a common experience for many Southeast Asian refugees and early Chinese immigrants. Adjustment to the United States for these groups often includes lifelong reactions to issues of separation, loss, and abandonment guilt. Coupled with a lack of familiarity with Western systems of care, many immigrants and refugees tend to underutilize health care services, delay seeking health care, show poor adherence, and experience barriers to quality health care.

By Westerners Toward Asians

The perception by Westerners of Asians as exotic, primitive, subservient, and passive results in bias within the health care system. Viewed as non-complaining or passive or perceived as a model minority, there is a tendency to overlook or ignore health disparities among Asian Americans. This is compounded by the absence of meaningful data on Asian American health status in most public health databases because of inadequate sampling. The resulting message is often that it is unnecessary or unimportant to attend to the unique health care needs of Asian Americans (5).

World-Views

Different world-views between Westerners and Asians exist in their orientation to nature and the environment, approaches to movement in space, and use of language. Orientation here relates to conceptualizations of time, space, and causality. These world-views influence the practice of health behaviors and attitudes toward health and health care delivery.

The philosophical *Zeitgeist* of most Asian cultures has been described as a combination of fatalistic and deterministic beliefs, of most Western cultures as a combination of deterministic and free will beliefs. Values of Asian and Asian American cultures reflect an emphasis on group orientation, collectivism, and interdependence versus Western emphasis on person orientation, individualism, and independence. Similarly there is an emphasis in Asian cultures on cooperation and harmony over competition and mastery. Social relationships emphasize and value those with authority figures based on duty, obligation, and self-discipline, and tend to be formal compared with Western emphasis on free will, personal rights, and a more informal and spontaneous communication style. Asian attitudes tend to be more pessimistic than optimistic and communication more often indirect than direct (6).

The use of language also differs between Asian and Western cultures. Culturally specific communications are apparent in the tendency and value placed on concise and indirect communication. In writing, brevity is valued as an indication of scholarship; emphasis is placed on the use of metaphor and nuances in meaning. Whereas Western values stress getting one's point across, Asian values stress politeness in verbal discourse. As a result, Westerners typically value verbal fluency, whereas Asians typically value not showing overt disagreement. Asian cultures, defined as *high-context cultures,* rely more on nonverbal context for information than on verbal context (7). Asians are commonly known to resort to indirect methods to communicate their intent and have developed the use of indirect communication to an art form. These differences explain the common phenomenon experienced by physicians in whom silence or head nodding is interpreted as agreement when the patient is merely being polite so as not to offend or embarrass the physician.

These orientations are also reflected in differences between the practice of Western and Asian medicine. Western models of study emphasize counting, empirical methods, and objectivity (i.e., science); consequently, Western medical tradition emphasizes dissection, analysis, and the use of diagnostic tools to detect disease. In contrast, the reliance on spirituality and philosophy within Asian methods of healing has been viewed by Westerners as phenomenologic, unscientific, and unproven. Asian methods are often at odds with those emphasized in Western methods of health care. For Asians, the emphasis on a holistic approach to the environment carries over to its healing methods of linking mind, body, and soul. The practice of Asian medicine emphasizes revitalizing body functions, maintaining balance, and restoring the body to its natural condition in its environment versus the Western practice of eradicating the germ, parasite, or pain (8).

Many Asian Americans incorporate these traditional views and beliefs in their health behaviors and may use culturally syntonic methods (e.g., herbal medicine, acupuncture) while simultaneously using Western medicine. On the other hand, however, Asian healing methods are usually not available or valued as quality care within the Western health care delivery system.

Health Beliefs

Although the use of Asian healing methods may be more common among immigrants and refugees, health beliefs common to Asians continue to influence the health behaviors and lifestyles of many Asian Americans.

Concepts of Health

Health must embrace a holistic view of well-being; health is a dynamic relationship focused on physical, social, psychological, and spiritual well-being. According to most Asian cultures, the balance of the *yin* and *yang* qualities in the body is considered critical to good health and well-being. These qualities represent opposites (female and male, cold and hot, earth and heaven). For example, Asian cultures hold that foods have "hot" and "cold" properties (*yang* and *yin*) and associate these with the nutritional qualities, medicinal value, and healing power of most foods.

Basic essences of the body include *qi* (breath, wind, or respiratory energy), blood which helps to produce *qi* while *qi* moves the blood, *jing* (essence including reproductive hormones and semen), and *shen* (spirit related to the heart and emotional conditions, body fluids). Pathological conditions of *qi* (wind) or the five basic elements of nature (water, earth, fire, metal, and wood) cause illness. Excess or deficiencies of moisture or toxins cause symptoms. For example, deficiencies of *yin* give rise to symptoms of dryness (e.g., dry mouth, cough) and heat (e.g., fever, inflammation), whereas deficiencies of *yang* give rise to symptoms of poor vitality and strength (e.g., fatigue, impotence) and lack of adequate warmth (e.g., chills). Wind usually attacks the upper part of the body (e.g., respiratory tract) so Asians avoid sitting near an air conditioner or in front of a fan. Dampness (e.g., getting caught in the rain, having wet hair, keeping on wet clothes, drinking too many cold drinks) is associated with symptoms of lethargy, indigestion, nausea, vomiting, or believed to cause arthritis.

Failure of these essences to regulate one another or external trauma (e.g., surgery) is viewed as a deficiency that causes the body to become imbalanced or interrupts the flow of *qi* such that blood circulates poorly or is obstructed. The belief is that cold causes the arteries to constrict in order to conserve heat, and disturbs the *qi* flow, causing "wind pain", chronic muscle spasms, and headaches. Not enough heat or fire in the body causes weakness; too much heat causes fever or cold sores.

Ayurveda

Asian Indians have a holistic system of healing, *ayurveda* ("science of life"), that originated more than 3000 years ago with the Brahmin sages. Several aspects of this system of medicine distinguish it from other approaches to health care. The focus is on establishing and maintaining balance of the life energies within the individual, rather than focusing on particular symptoms. *Ayurveda* recognizes that each individual has a unique constitution; therefore prevention and treatment regimens are based on the individual, not on illness, disease, or symptom. It also recognizes the total connection between the mind and body and between the individual and nature. *Ayurveda* identifies three basic types of energy or functional principles that are present in everyone and everything. The Sanskrit words for these basic energies are *vata, pitta,* and *kapha.* These principles can be related to the basic biology of the body (9,10).

Wellness versus Illness

Whether patients define themselves as sick (of "ill-health") may be related to Asian health beliefs. Illness may be denied or attributed to personal carelessness or weakness, viewed as punishment, or considered a result of external forces over which the patient has no control. Physicians, on the other hand, may attribute illness to diet, genetics, or other biological processes. Sometimes patient denial is associated with economic factors (e.g., the need to keep working) or social factors (e.g., the inability to ask for help). Popular practices for maintaining health and restoring the balance of body essences are thus distinguished from medical care necessary to eradicate acute conditions of illness. Many Asian Americans will simultaneously practice Asian and Western healing methods or resort to the other when one fails. It is when these beliefs contradict one another that poor compliance with Western medicine is likely to occur.

Asians often view Western medicine, based as it seems on pills and surgery, as external assaults on the body. Eastern medicine, in contrast, is seen as attempting to regulate and correct internal body states and conditions. Acupuncture and herbal medicine can restore the balance of body essences, or the *yin/yang* qualities of the body. Also necessary are a nutritional diet and appropriate lifestyle behaviors to maintain wellness and longevity. Western medicine is often viewed as more powerful for acute conditions of illness, whereas Eastern medicine is viewed as essential to regulating daily health functioning. When Western medicine fails, patients resort to Eastern medicine.

Causation of Illness

Cultural concepts of free will and fate are integral to health beliefs about the cause of illness. Fatalistic views of the world, common among Asians, often lead to resignation when faced with major illness or genetic conditions. It is not uncommon for parents to view the birth of a child with a birth defect or with cognitive impairment as one's fate or as causally linked to some event in the past ranging from the mystical to the concrete. Consequently, many health behaviors are practiced to avoid adverse consequences. Pregnant women are careful to avoid foods with too much *yang* quality, for example.

Religion and Spirituality

Spiritualism in Asian cultures is often linked to Confucianism, Buddhism, Taoism, or Shinto. Confucianism, considered a philosophy rather than a religion, speaks to social order and defines the relationship of authority and hierarchy, and is conceived to produce a harmonious balance of obligations in interpersonal relationships. In Confucian doctrine the Emperor was at the center of earthly power, who showed by example the proper forms of filial worship of ancestors and the wise governance of his own family. The daily workings of government, however, were delegated to the learned men and scholars who would rule wisely.

Taoism derived from the subordinate orders and found its way into popular literature as a way of criticizing the Confucian order that ruled society. Taoists used literature to publicize the crimes of the mighty and the injustices suffered by the subordinates including women, children, and even animals. As critics of the social order, they often joined the peasants in resisting and overthrowing the dynasty in power, thus translating their egalitarian view of creation into social and economic reality (11). Whereas Confucianism emphasized hierarchical relationships in the social order and the dominance of males over females, Taoism emphasized egalitarianism in these relationships. These opposing doctrines, Confucianism and Taoism, gave shape to Chinese culture and to this day influence views of any social system including the health care system.

Buddhism, on the other hand, emphasizes respect and enlightenment, and attaining an understanding of the universe. Buddhism is often considered an educational system rather than a religion, because the Buddha is not a supernatural being but rather someone who has achieved this complete understanding (12). With the view that human suffering is the plight of mankind, healing does not emphasize the absence of pain as it does in Western medicine. For this reason, one is likely to encounter higher levels of pain tolerance among Asians with strong Buddhist beliefs.

A connecting concept between Taoism and Buddhism is that the spirits of the dead may reappear in animal form to atone for the sins of previous lifetimes. Beliefs in demons and/or ancestral spirits causing or influencing ill health are common and reflect a sense of generational connectivity and continuity of the present life with the afterlife. Spirits are often said to visit one's dreams. These beliefs may cause or increase feelings of hopelessness when a patient is faced with major illness. Clinicians should therefore consider and acknowledge such beliefs when informing patients about life-threatening diagnoses and when discussing issues of death and dying.

Shinto is a religion native to Japan, characterized by veneration of nature spirits and ancestors. It has no written scripture or body of religious law.

Some Asians have adopted Christianity as their faith, with Catholicism and Protestantism often serving as the backdrop for Confucian doctrine. Catholicism has been embraced by Koreans, in particular. Other religions practiced by Asians include Islam (particularly among South Asians) and Hinduism.

Health and Lifestyle Behaviors

Exercise

Emphasis on lifestyle behaviors is a fairly recent phenomenon caused by the increase in leisure time as a result of technological advances and the decrease in mortality from infectious disease. At the same time, emphasis on a daily regimen of health behaviors and exercise has been common in Asian cultures, consistent with a holistic view of mind, body, and spirit as important to health and wellness. Tai Chi, a form of exercise, and Qi Gong, the development of internal energy, are viewed as supportive of longevity, health, and strength. The former involves slow movements of the body that stimulate and exercise internal parts of the body; the latter combines breathing control, relaxation, meditation, and martial arts to achieve calmness and feeling centered or to develop stamina and strength. These traditional forms of exercise have been practiced for centuries to promote health, build resiliency, and improve circulation of body essences. Among early Asian American immigrants, these behaviors went into decline because of the rigorous demands of economic conditions and work schedules. Recognition of the shift toward volitional forms of exercise is important.

Diet

Asian diets are often designed to treat many ailments and to maintain balance of *yin/yang* properties in the body. Consequently, herbal soups and tonics are commonly used to restore or maintain health and well-being. This contrasts with dieting in the Western context, which is mostly intended to reduce weight, although Asian practices (e.g., the use of ginseng, ginkgo nuts, and other herbal tonics associated with health-restoring properties) are increasingly being adopted by Westerners. Depending on the presence of symptoms, diets may be altered or tonics prepared to restore *yin/yang* balances. Foods such as black pepper, ginger, yam, longan, and garlic are considered high in *yang* properties, whereas foods such as seaweed, tomato, kidney, lettuce, and liver are considered high in *yin* properties (13).

Recommendations to a patient of Asian background for diet modification or exercise to address high cholesterol and hypertension, for example, and chronic disease prevention and management are more likely to be followed if concepts of Asian dietary practice are taken into account. For examples of Asian food pyramids, visit the Web site of the Southeastern Michigan Dietetic Association (www.semda.org).

Social and Family Structure

Stress and quality-of-life issues are being increasingly emphasized as rapid transformation of society occurs through advances in technology and longer lifespan. Coping with chronic disease has taken precedence over struggles to fight infectious disease, starvation, and malnutrition. While many Asian immigrants came to the United States to escape poverty, starvation, and disease, they often retain coping mechanisms that are no longer needed. Yet, these continue to influence the psychosocial adjustment and views of health among many Asian American immigrants.

An extended family structure has been an important social pattern within most Asian communities. Enclaves of ethnic concentrations in the form of Chinatowns, Japantowns, and Koreatowns that recreate social and community systems of support left behind in the countries of origin are common among many Asian American immigrant and refugee groups. These are most visibly organized around food and restaurants but also around religion (common among Korean Americans) and language schools (common among Chinese Americans). It is not uncommon for social structures to be organized around family clans.

These social structures also sustain lifestyle behaviors that affect health. For example, smoking is common among immigrant male restaurant workers as a social pastime, with rates exceeding 50%. Tai Chi is a common shared activity among the elderly.

Gender roles within Asian American groups are complex and often erroneously interpreted. Though Confucian philosophy promulgated male-dominant cultures, opportunities for connectedness existed in agrarian cultures of communes where women worked side by side with men and in family circles where women were dominant in governing the household. Gender issues among Asian Americans have often been secondary to issues of culture and race given the sociopolitical context of the United States. Discussion of how these roles have evolved can be found elsewhere (14). However, not unlike in Western cultures, Asian women are often those responsible for health care decisions. They sustain rituals related to health, for example, preparing herbal tonics and medicinal soups to restore health following childbirth or surgery.

Major Health Concerns for Asian Americans

How Asian Americans view health and illness is only one aspect of cultural difference in the practice of cross-cultural medicine. Increasingly, the literature suggests that race and ethnicity contribute significantly to different manifestations of disease and differences in health status. Furthermore, perception of Asian cultures as exotic, primitive, subservient, and passive by Westerners may result in bias within the health care system. Also, because Asian Americans are sometimes viewed as a "model minority", there is a tendency to overlook health disparities in this population. Disparities in health status between white and minority racial and ethnic groups exist despite federal initiatives to eliminate them.

This situation is compounded by the absence of meaningful data on Asian American health status in most public health databases. Many studies fail to show statistically significant differences in morbidity and mortality between Asian Americans and whites, whereas others show Asian Americans to be in better health than white Americans. Asians are often considered too few to be counted as a separate group; they are often omitted or counted as "other" in public health datasets. Even when Asians are included, failure to disaggregate data by ethnic groups often masks significant differences among the diverse Asian American groups. Recommendations for methodological changes such as oversampling, using qualitative and ethnographic data, and re-analysis have yet to be implemented (15).

The 1985 Heckler Report (16) on black and minority health clearly demonstrated excess morbidity and mortality directly related to social inequalities but at the same time perpetuated the "model minority" myth about Asian Americans. Asian Americans were considered to be in good health because the report failed to include a sufficient sample to do meaningful analyses and did not include health conditions (e.g., tuberculosis and hepatitis B) prevalent among Asian American populations. The limited studies that have been undertaken on Asian American health are often published in non-peer reviewed journals because mainstream journals consider them of "limited scope and relevance".

In general, Asian Americans are subject to many of the same health problems as other racial and ethnic groups. Studies that have specifically studied Asian Americans have identified meaningful differences in the major health conditions of diabetes, cancer, and cardiovascular disease when the data are disaggregated (17).

Cancer

King and Locke (18) note there has been a downward transition for cancers with high risk among Asian Chinese and an upward displacement for cancers of low risk for Foshan and Hong Kong Chinese following migration to the United States. These trends suggest that environmental factors are implicated with a "gradient" in which behaviors and characteristics (e.g., diet, smoking, acculturation, other socioeconomic factors) change as individuals move from one country to another (19). Migrant studies comparing groups in their country of origin with immigrants from that country in the United States show that alterations in cancer rates move toward patterns in the country of adoption and are probably due to environmental and lifestyle changes such as diet and cigarette smoking (20).

Higher rates of different and site-specific cancers have been found. Chinese males show an excess incidence of nasopharyngeal, esophageal, stomach, gallbladder, and liver cancer. Liver cancer rates are higher in male Chinese, Japanese, and Filipino immigrants than in American-born Asian men (21).

Asian American women in general have lower rates of breast cancer deaths than white American women, though their rates in the United States are higher than the rates prevailing in Asia (22). The high rate of soy product use among women living in Asia may account for some of the observed difference in breast cancer incidence. Mammography screening rates are low among Asian American women, and Asian women born outside the United States are more likely to present with breast cancers that are greater than 1 cm (23). Vietnamese and Korean American women have higher rates of cervical cancer than the general American population. Screening for cervical cancer among some Asian American women is low; in some studies nearly half of Asian women have never had a Pap smear. Lack of familiarity with the Pap test is a major barrier to screening (24).

Diabetes

The prevalence of diabetes mellitus is increasing in the general United States population but is increasing more rapidly among Asian Americans (increasing 10% to 15% among Asian Americans between 1990 and 1998 compared with 5% among whites) (25). Previous studies of Japanese Americans in Seattle and Hawaii showed the prevalence of diabetes was two to three times higher than in Japan. The prevalence of diabetes among Chinese Americans is five to seven times higher than in China.

Little is known about the long-term complications and risk factors for diabetes among Asian Americans (26). Type 2, or non-insulin dependent, diabetes accounts for almost all cases of diabetes in Asian American populations. Whereas the prevalence of obesity and diabetes has been correlated for Pacific Islanders (i.e., Samoans and Native Hawaiians), it is less true for other Asian American groups in which obesity based on body mass indices is a poorer predictor of the risk for diabetes (27,28). The criterion for obesity among Asian Americans has been defined as a BMI of 25 compared with a definition of 30 for whites. Asian Indians have significantly higher rates of gestational diabetes, insulin resistance, and centripetal obesity (29), all of which are associated with the development of type 2 diabetes.

Cardiovascular Disease

Coronary heart disease and stroke are the leading causes of deaths for most racial and ethnic groups in the United States. Coronary heart disease deaths are lower among Chinese and Japanese Americans than among African Americans and whites. Deaths from stroke are proportionally higher than deaths from coronary heart disease among Japanese and Chinese Americans. Conversely, deaths from coronary heart disease are proportionally higher than deaths from stroke among Asian Indians (30). The risk of coronary heart disease among Asian Indians is not explained by high cholesterol, cigarette smoking, and hypertension but by levels of lipoprotein alpha-1, an independent risk factor for premature atherosclerosis that is disproportionately elevated in Asian Indians (31). Acute myocardial infarction is more prevalent among Indians who have immigrated to the West or who live in urban centers in India; the increased risk is thought to be due to changes in lifestyle that lead to weight gain and dietary changes (32). Although South Asians use large quantities of vegetables in their traditional cooking, the use of coconut oils and *ghee* (clarified butter) increases fat content and contributes to the risk of heart disease.

Hepatitis

Although the prevalence of the hepatitis B carrier state is relatively low in the United States (0.1% to 2% of the population), the prevalence among immigrants is higher. As mentioned earlier, more than 50% of Asian Americans are foreign born. The prevalence of hepatitis B chronic carriers among Asian Americans is between 8% and 15% (32a). Asian Americans make up almost 50% of all chronic carriers in the United States. The majority of Asian Americans acquired infection at birth via perinatal transmission (33). Rates of hepatitis B range from 3% to 5% in intermediate prevalence areas (e.g., Japan and Central Asia) to 10% to 20% in high prevalence areas (e.g., Southeast Asia and China). Asian Americans from these areas should be screened for hepatitis B and vaccinated as appropriate. Pregnant Asian-born women should be screened and their infants vaccinated. One study found that 8% of Asian American pregnant women were positive for hepatitis B surface antigen; another study reports a prevalence of 12% to 14% among Southeast Asian immigrants (34). Hepatitis B infection is a major cause of liver cancer among Asian Americans.

Tuberculosis

The tuberculosis incidence rate is five times greater among Asian Americans than in the general United States population (35). Tuberculosis in foreign-born persons residing in the United States represents nearly 42% of all TB diagnoses in the United States. Immigrants from Mexico, the Philippines, Vietnam, India, China, Haiti, and South Korea were responsible for approximately two-thirds of foreign-born cases (36). Nearly one-half of tuberculosis cases among immigrants occur more than five years after arrival in the

United States. The incidence of resistance to isoniazide was 11.6% and to both isoniazide and rifampin was 1.7% in one recent report (37). Physicians should be aware of appropriate screening, diagnosis, and treatment guidelines for TB.

Reproductive Health

Asian women generally have excellent birth outcomes, with low infant mortality rates. However, the percentage of low birthweight babies varies substantially among Asian groups, with Vietnamese, Cambodian, Filipino, and Asian Indian American women having the highest rates of low birthweight infants (38-40). Asian American women experience menopause differently than other women. Many women do not experience any symptoms associated with the cessation of their menstrual periods (41). In some Asian languages there is no comparable word for menopause.

Modesty is an important factor for many Asian American women and may present a barrier to obtaining prenatal care and cervical and breast cancer screening if female clinicians are not available (42). However, physicians should not make assumptions about the attitude that Asian women may have toward clinical examinations (Case 5-1).

Mental Health

Mental health problems are prevalent among Asian Americans, although they often exhibit culturally distinct symptoms and different manifestations compared with white Americans (43). Concepts of mental health vary among different Asiatic groups, making exploration of mental health problems, diagnosis, and treatment a challenge.

Often Asian American mental health problems are associated with somatic complaints. The terms for mental health problems reflect the correlation between the mind and the body. For example, in the Chinese language the term for depression is associated with the heart. Patients with depression often present with headaches, dizziness, heart palpitations, or stomach pain. These symptoms are not a denial of depression but rather a manifestation of it. Failure to understand this presentation can lead to misdiagnosis. Suicide rates among Asians are lower than for whites, but Native Hawaiian adolescents, young women immigrants from India, and Asian American women over 65 have the highest risk among Asians and Pacific Islanders (44).

CASE 5-1   A 37-YEAR-OLD ASIAN INDIAN WOMAN WHO APPEARS UNCOMFORTABLE DURING GYNECOLOGIC EXAMINATION

MM is a 37-year-old Asian Indian woman who has recently moved to the United States. She has never had a Pap smear. After careful discussion with her physician, she agrees to have a pelvic examination and Pap smear. Before the examination, as the physician is assisting her into the footrests, the physician notes that she appears quite uncomfortable. Assuming that she is nervous regarding the pelvic examination, the physician stops to discuss the matter with her. The patient says that she is not nervous about the examination ("I've had two children and that does not bother me") but that in her country touching others with your feet is a sign of disrespect. She was uncomfortable when the physician handled her feet because she did not want to demean her physician. The physician thanks her for the explanation and allows the patient to place her own feet in the stirrups. The examination proceeds without problem.

DISCUSSION

In this case the physician made the assumption that the patient's distress was caused by embarrassment or nervousness regarding the pelvic examination. But her distress was due to a particular cultural value that she felt was violated. By talking with the patient and recognizing her cultural values, the provider avoided an awkward situation.

Asian Americans tend to underutilize mental health services (45) and often are reluctant to seek help for mental health problems because of language and cultural barriers (46). Stigma and shame over using services, lack of financial resources, concepts about mental health and services that differ from Western concepts, cultural inappropriateness of services, and use of folk healers are some reasons for this underutilization. In Western cultures, depression is a psychiatric syndrome with specific affective, cognitive, behavioral, and somatic symptoms. In many Asian cultures, there is no equivalent concept of depression (47). Asian Americans commonly seek treatment through primary care, where they can focus on their physical symptoms and under-report emotional symptoms (48).

Many Southeast Asian immigrants have had histories of trauma associated with war, resulting in a high incidence of post-traumatic stress disorders (PTSDs). Symptoms of PTSD differ among Asian immigrants. For example, blindness is a common problem among Cambodian women while flashbacks are largely absent. Symptoms can persist for many years after arrival in the United States (49). Adjustment to the United States for these individuals often includes lifelong reactions to separation, loss, and abandonment guilt.

Pharmacologic Considerations

There is growing evidence of differential responses to some medications among Asian Americans. Propranolol has a greater effect on blood pressure and heart rate in Chinese than in whites (50). Differences in metabolism and clinical outcomes have also been demonstrated for metoprolol, enalapril, and amitriptyline. These differences result in a greater response to a given medicine and more side effects (Case 5-2) (51).

Attitudes Towards Terminal Illness

In the United States ethical principles of autonomy, beneficence, and veracity are imbedded in clinical settings and in the doctor-patient interaction. Several studies have demonstrated, however, that all racial or ethnic groups do not share these principles (52). Some Asian families believe that sharing cancer diagnoses and poor prognoses with patients is not appropriate and that family members should be the ones to make decisions about treatment options and the use of life support. Physicians should therefore explore choices with patients and their families *before* the occasion arises (53). Physicians should not make assumptions about how an elderly Asian American would feel about this situation, however, as is illustrated in Case 5-3.

Barriers to Access to Care

Immigrant and refugee populations typically face poor access to health care because of language, cultural, and financial barriers. Because more than half of Asian Americans are foreign born, access to care is a major concern. The

CASE 5-2   A 72-YEAR-OLD MAN OF CHINESE DESCENT WHO DOES NOT COMPLY WITH PRESCRIBED TREATMENT

MC is a 72-year-old man of Chinese descent. He immigrated to the United States in 1980 and worked as a technologist in a research laboratory until his recent retirement. He has hypertension, which has not been well controlled. His physician prescribed atenolol 50 mg daily the last time he was seen.

At follow-up the patient's blood pressure is 160/105, down from 170/110 two weeks ago, and his heart rate is 72. He tells the doctor he could not take all the atenolol and is only taking a half-tablet daily. He asks his doctor about adding a different medicine, a calcium channel blocking agent. After reviewing the patient's symptoms and examination results, his physician tells him that he should take the atenolol 50 mg daily because his heart rate is not too slow. The patient nods his head but does not intend to take the medicine as prescribed.

MC did not disclose during the office visit that he had experienced side effects from 50 mg of atenolol and found that 25 mg did not cause the same problems. He had conducted some research on antihypertensives and thought a calcium channel agent would be better. His internist is unaware that the patient was trained as a surgeon in China but never practiced in the United States.

DISCUSSION

This case illustrates several points. The patient demonstrates sensitivity to atenolol that is common among some Asians. He did not want to embarrass his physician by disagreeing with his assessment and refusing to take the higher dose. The physician could enhance his understanding of the patient and increase adherence to prescribed therapies by asking about the patient's perceptions of the problem (his explanatory model) and how he came to ask for a calcium channel blocker. Many physicians are unaware of the level of education or training of immigrants, and it is helpful to ask about this when completing a social history.

CASE 5-3   A 76-YEAR-OLD VIETNAMESE WOMAN WHO MAY OR MAY NOT BE DECLINING SURGERY

TL is a 76-year-old Vietnamese woman who has been receiving her primary care for three years from the same internist. After she complains of abdominal pain an evaluation reveals a large ovarian mass that is suspicious for a malignancy. Computed tomography detects no ascites, liver abnormalities, or other masses. A chest x-ray and liver and renal tests are normal. Her medical problems include hypertension, which is well controlled. She also has a past history of chest pain that was believed to be due to coronary artery disease. She is asymptomatic on atenolol and aspirin.

TL does not speak English and is usually accompanied to her appointments by her son, who interprets for her. The test results are described to the son and surgery is recommended. The son speaks with his mother. He then tells the physician that his mother will not have the surgery because she is too old and does not want it.

Two weeks later the patient and her son return for follow-up. The mother has lost a few pounds and continues to complain of abdominal discomfort. When the question of surgery is raised again, the son repeats that his mother is too old for surgery.

DISCUSSION

The major problem in this case is that the primary care provider does not know what the son has told his mother and whether he is the one making the decision that his mother is too old for surgery. While scheduling follow-up, the physician has a good opportunity to ask the son to bring in other important members of the family to have a discussion. Most importantly, the physician should schedule a Vietnamese interpreter to be present when all the information is reviewed to ensure that the patient has an opportunity to participate in her own care if so desired.

In this case a meeting took place with a skilled medical interpreter, the patient, and her son, granddaughter, and daughter-in-law. The patient decided that she wanted to have the surgery, which was successful in that her abdominal discomfort resolved. Her ovarian mass was benign.

absence of or limited supply of interpreters and bilingual providers impedes access and communication. Even when interpreters are available, the multiple dialects and languages among different Asian ethnic groups make communication difficult. Poverty, lack of insurance, limited education, cultural views of hospitals as a place to die, and mistrust and unfamiliarity with Western health care systems result in delayed care and low use of available facilities and programs.

Bipolar distributions on these factors tend to mask the large numbers of non-English speaking, poor, and uninsured Asian Americans. In 1990, 82% of Asian Americans and Pacific Islanders 25 years or older had four years of high school education, but the percentage who had less than a fifth grade education was greater than 5%, which is nearly twice that of the general United States population. The median family income for Asian Americans and Pacific Islanders was higher than for the total population, but the percentage who live in poverty is higher than for the general population (4). Poverty levels tend to be higher among Southeast Asians, Samoans, and Cantonese Chinese immigrant groups. In one study, 27% of Asians were uninsured compared with 12% of whites, 19% of blacks, and 27% of Hispanics (54). Patients often need to access care through complicated telephone systems that are unresponsive to non-English speakers. Longer waits for services occur when interpreters cannot be found or child family members are called upon to interpret.

Moreover, the inability or lack of responsiveness by providers to different cultural beliefs, values, and practices often compromises the quality of the care that is delivered. Most health care systems cannot identify the ethnicity of their providers if a client seeks a provider who is ethnically similar or culturally competent. Given the subtle but significant differences in communication patterns, health-seeking behaviors, views of health, and health status, quality of care is compromised when services are not culturally competent (55,56).

Cross-Cultural Applications

The patterns and trends common among Asian Americans are not intended as stereotypic prescriptions; rather they are intended to illustrate significant and unique differences in health behavior, beliefs, and epidemiology that will influence health care utilization and health status. When patients and physicians come from different cultures, physicians need to learn both the latest findings on specific ethnic health risks and the best skills for effective cross-cultural communication.

Risk Management

Physicians who make diagnoses based on the "typical" diseases found among the general population may misdiagnose if they do not consider or are not aware of specific ethnic health risks and responses to illness, utilization, compliance, and behaviors.

Enhancing Medical Compliance

Out of politeness or respect for authority, an Asian American patient may not communicate his disagreement with the medical recommendations of his health care provider. For example, whereas Westerners believe a cool bath should be used to bring down a fever, Asians believe that keeping one warm with blankets following the use of a herbal tea will dissipate fever. Consequently, there is a likelihood of noncompliance with recommendations about treating fevers.

Asians often believe that blood is not replenished when removed from the body. Thus the Asian American patient may be reluctant to have blood drawn and may need reassurance that it is safe and not harmful and that only the minimum amount necessary for the test will be drawn.

Physicians using Western paradigms of the *body* as distinct from the *mind* and *soul* may experience poor empathic relationships with their clients. They may fail to understand the manifestations of symptoms in their Asian American clients who may describe their somatic symptoms in relation to other dimensions (e.g., fate, spiritual and cosmic influences). Or they may view these beliefs as superstition. Not knowing the use of indirect communication, they may misunderstand silence, face resistance to their recommendations, or not understand the need to ask facilitative questions. Without cross-cultural communication, there is likely to be struggle, mistrust, or poor compliance in the patient-provider encounter.

Integrating Sociopolitical Contexts into the Clinical Encounter

Physicians ignorant of the sociopolitical context of patient experiences may misinterpret behaviors and make inappropriate recommendations. They may misunderstand behaviors used adaptively in past situations and deem the patient resistant, hostile, or mistrustful. For example, patients who have experienced detention camps are less likely to be forthcoming during history taking or willing to reveal information for fear of retribution.

Respecting Cultural Health Beliefs

As we have discussed, cultural health beliefs encompass not only beliefs regarding disease and its causation but also attitudes about the maintenance of health itself. Clinicians should be aware of and respect these beliefs. For example, physicians who are unaware of cultural and spiritual beliefs about death and dying may inadvertently trigger an individual and family crisis by not conforming to social rules about approaching taboo subjects. Discussing customs about who makes health care decisions, and deciding how and if an individual should be told about a life-threatening diagnosis, must be handled delicately with a respect for the client's belief system.

Providers should bear in mind that Asian health practices such as acupuncture and herbal medicine are often used in tandem with Western medicine. If a patient reports using such Asian healing methods, the physician should ask about what other health measures the patient is taking, rather than make assumptions.

Conclusion

The medical care of Asian Americans will be effective only if it is culturally competent. When providers and patients have differing cultural perspectives, it is incumbent on the provider not only to understand the specific culture of the patient but also to learn skills for effective cross-cultural communication and to ensure a framework for avoiding bias in diagnosis and treatment. The world-views and values of Asian and Western cultures differ greatly in many areas. However, although these differences have historically formed the basis for mutual misunderstanding and mistrust, an empathetic patient-physician relationship can be created when care is delivered in a culturally competent fashion. Culturally competent care means that providers and all levels of a health care delivery system are able to address the needs of specific communities and incorporate cultural beliefs, values, and practices in the delivery of health care.

Summary of Asian Views on Health

- Emphasis on holism
- Links mind, body, and soul
- Balance is important (*yin/yang*)
- Basic essences of the body
  - Breath or wind (*qi*)
  - Blood
  - Reproductive hormones, semen (*jing*)
  - Spirit (*shen*)
- Ancestral spirits can cause or influence ill health
- *Ayurveda*
  - Holistic system of healing established by Brahmin sages of India
  - Focus on establishing and maintaining balance of life energies within
  - Each individual has a unique constitution
  - Prevention and treatment based on individual constitution, not symptoms
- Use of Asian and Western medicine simultaneously is common

Summary of Obstacles to Health Care Delivery to Asian Americans

- Absence or limited supply of qualified interpreters and bilingual providers
  - >50% of Asian Americans are foreign born
  - Accessing care often involves using complicated telephone systems ("menus") that are not understood by non-English-speaking persons
  - Limited translated materials
- Immigrants and refugees experience higher rates of
  1) Poverty
     - The percentage of certain Asian American groups who live in poverty is higher than for the general United States population
  2) Lack of health insurance
     - 27% of Asians versus 12% of whites do not have health insurance
  3) Limited education
     - 5% of Asian Americans have less than a 5th grade education (almost twice the percentage in the general population)
- Mistrust of Western medicine
- Cultural views and health behaviors often are inconsistent with those supported by Western medicine
- Health care systems often fail to integrate cultural factors into their delivery of care

Summary of High-Risk Conditions and Other Health Issues in Asians and Asian Americans

Be on the alert for presenting signs of the following conditions. Keep in mind that the history-taking must take into account cultural differences that may otherwise mislead the physician (e.g., reluctance to discuss psychological problems).

High-Risk Conditions

- Cancer
  - ◆ Cancer rates for Asians increase after immigration to the United States
  - ◆ Increased incidence of the following (among men):
    - ➤ Nasopharyngeal cancer
    - ➤ Esophageal cancer
    - ➤ Stomach cancer
    - ➤ Gallbladder cancer
    - ➤ Liver cancer
  - ◆ Cervical cancer incidence especially high in Southeast Asian and Korean women
- Type 2 diabetes
  - ◆ Occurs at lower BMI
- Cardiovascular disease (including hypertension)
  - ◆ Especially among Asian Indians
- Hepatitis B
  - ◆ Asian Americans constitute 50% of all chronic carriers in the United States
  - ◆ Most Asian Americans with hepatitis B acquired infection at birth via perinatal transmission; pregnant Asian-born women should be screened and their infants vaccinated
- Tuberculosis
  - ◆ Tuberculosis rate for Asians is five times greater than for the general population
- Post-traumatic stress disorders and depression, especially among Southeast Asians

Pharmacologic Considerations

Some drugs are metabolized differently in Asian Americans than in the general population (e.g., metoprolol, enalapril, amitriptyline).

Other Considerations

- Prevalence rates among Asian Americans are lower for breast cancer.
- Menopause is often not accompanied by symptoms.

Summary of Communication Issues in Caring for Asian Americans

- In general, brevity is valued by Asian Americans.
- Indirect rather than direct communication tends to be used.
- Use of metaphors and nuance is common.
- Asians stress politeness, even in disagreement, and therefore may appear to agree with a treatment plan when in fact they may not intend to comply with it.

REFERENCES

1. Barnes JS, Bennett CE. The Asian Population: Census 2000 Brief. Washington, DC: Census Bureau; February 2002.
2. Williams HC. Have you ever seen an Asian/Pacific Islander? Arch Dermatol. 2002;138: 673-4.
3. Takaki R. Strangers from a Different Shore. Boston: Little, Brown; 1987.
4. Lin-Fu JS. Asian and Pacific Islander Americans: an overview of demographic characteristics and health care issues. Asian American and Pacific Islander Journal of Health. 1993;1:20-35.
5. Yoon E, Chien F. Asian American and Pacific Islander health: a paradigm for minority health. JAMA. 1996;275:736-8.
6. Kawahara Y. Cultural value orientations of Asian Americans and European Americans, personal communication, 1997.
7. Chin JL, Liem JH, Hong G, Ham M. Transference and empathy in Asian Americans, personal communication, 1993.
8. Kim MC. Oriental medicine and cancer. Belmont, MA: Seven Galaxy Publications; 1996:12.
9. Lad V. Ayurveda: A Brief Introduction and Guide. Albuquerque, NM: The Ayurvedic Institute; 1996.
10. Shama HM, Brihaspati DT, Chopra D. Maharashi Ayur-veda: modern insights into ancient medicine. JAMA. 1991;272:2633-7.
11. Roberts M. Chinese fairy-tales and fantasies. New York: Pantheon; 1979.
12. King VMC. A path to true happiness. Richardson, TX: Dallas Buddhist Association; 1998.
13. Lu HC. Chinese system of food cures: prevention and remedies. New York: Sterling Publishing; 1986.
14. Chin JL. Relationships among Asian American women. Washington, DC: American Psychological Association; 2000.
15. Yu E. Methodological issues. In: Zane NWS, Takeuchi DT, Young KNJ (eds). Confronting Critical Health Issues of Asian and Pacific Islander Women. Thousand Oaks, CA: Sage Publications; 1994:22-50.
16. Report of the Secretary's Task Force on Black and Minority Health. Vol 1. Executive Summary. Washington, DC: Department of Health and Human Services; 1985.

17. Chin JL. Asian American health in Massachusetts: myth and facts. Asian American and Pacific Islander Journal of Health. 1999;7:150-64.

18. King H, Locke FB. Health effects of migration: U.S. Chinese in and outside the China-town. International Migration Review. 1987;21:555-75.

19. Gardner R. Mortality. In: Confronting Critical Health Issues of Asian and Pacific Islander Women. Thousand Oaks, CA: Sage Publications; 1994:53-104.

20. Li FP, Pawlish K. Cancers in Asian Americans and Pacific Islanders: migrant studies. Asian American and Pacific Islander Journal of Health. 1998;6:123-9.

21. Rosenblatt KA, Weiss NS, Schwartz SM. Liver cancer in Asian migrants to the United States and their descendents. Cancer Causes Control. 1996;7:345-50.

22. Wu AH, Ziegler RG, Horn-Ross PL, et al. Tofu and risk of breast cancer in Asian-Americans. Cancer Epidemiol Biomarkers Prev. 1996;5:901-6.

23. Ashley H, White E, Taylor V. Ethnicity and birthplace in relation to tumor size and stage in Asian American women with breast cancer. Am J Pub Health. 1999;89:1248-52.

24. Kim K, Yu E, Chen EH, et al. Cervical cancer screening knowledge and practices among Korean American women. Cancer Nursing. 1999;22:297-302.

25. Joslin Diabetes Center. Asian American Diabetes Fund Newsletter. 2002; vol 1.

26. Smith FE, Chiu JL, King GL. Diabetes mellitus and its complications in Asian Americans. Asian American and Pacific Islander Journal of Health. 1999;7:170-5.

27. Fujimoto WY. Diabetes in Asian and Pacific Islander Americans. In: Harris M (ed). Diabetes in America. NIH Publication 95-1468. 1995:661-82.

28. King G, Joslin Diabetes Center, personal communication, 23 June 2000.

29. McKeigue PM, Shah B, Marmot MG. Relation of central obesity and insulin resistance with high diabetes prevalence and cardiovascular risk in South Asians. Lancet. 1991:337:382-6.

30. Wild SH, Laws A, Fortman SP, et al. Mortality from coronary heart disease and stroke for six ethnic groups in California, 1985-1990. Ann Epidemiol. 1995;5:432-9.

31. Pais P, Pogue J, Gerstein H, et al. Risk factors for acute myocardial infarction in Indians: a case-control study. Lancet. 1996;348:358-63.

32. Enas EA, Mehta J. Malignant coronary artery disease in young Asian Indians: thoughts on pathogenesis, prevention, and therapy. Coronary Artery Disease in Asian Indians (CADI) Study. Clin Cardiol. 1995;18:131-5.

32a. Hann HL. Hepatitis B. In: Zane NWS, Takeuchi DT, Young KNJ, eds. Confronting Critical Health Issues of Asian and Pacific Islander Americans. Thousand Oaks, CA: Sage Publications; 1994:148-69.

33. Stevens CE, Toy PT, Tong MJ, et al. Perinatal hepatitis B virus transmission in the United States: prevention by passive-active immunization. JAMA. 1985;253:1740-5.

34. Gjerdingen D, Lor V. Hepatitis B status among Hmong patients. J Am Board Fam Pract. 1997;10:322-8.

35. Tuberculosis among Asians and Pacific Islanders, U.S. 1985. MMWR. 1987;36:81.

36. McKenna MT, McCray E, Onorato I. The epidemiology of tuberculosis among foreign-born persons in the United States, 1986 to 1993. N Engl J Med. 1995;332:1071-6.

37. Talbot EA, Moore M, McCray E, Binkin NJ. Tuberculosis among foreign-born persons in the United States, 1993-1998. JAMA. 2000;284:2894-900.

38. Le LT, Liely JL, Schoendorf KC. Birthweight outcomes among Asian and Pacific Islander subgroups in the United Sates. Int J Epidemiol. 1996;25:973-9.

39. Singh GK, Yu SM. Birthweight differentials among Asian Americans. Am J Public Health. 1994;84:1444-9.

40. Fuentes-Afflick E, Hessol NA. Impact of Asian ethnicity and national origin on infant birth weight. Am J Epidemiol. 1997;145:148-55.

41. Bromberger JT, Meyer PM, Howard DO, et al. Psychologic distress and natural menopause: a multiethnic community study. Am J Public Health. 2001;91:1435-42.

42. Kelly AW, Chacori M, Wollan PC, et al. A program to increase breast and cervical cancer screening for Cambodian women in a Midwestern community. Mayo Clin Proc. 1996; 71:437-44.

43. Chun KM, Eastman KL, Wang GCS. Psychopathology. In: Lee LC, Zane NWS (eds). Handbook of Asian American Psychology. Thousand Oaks, CA: Sage Publications; 1998: 457-84.

44. Mental health care for Asian Americans and Pacific Islanders. In: Mental Health: Culture, Race, and Ethnicity. A Supplement to Mental Health: A Report of the Surgeon General. Rockville, MD: Department of Health and Human Services, Office of the Surgeon General; 2001:115.

45. Ying YW, Hu LT. Public outpatient mental health services: use and outcome among Asian Americans. Am J Orthopsychiatry. 1994;64:448-55.

46. Lin TY, Lin KM. Service delivery issues in Asian North American communities. Am J Psych. 1978;135:454-6.

47. Marsella AJ, Sartorius N, Jablensky A, Fenton FR. Cross-cultural studies of depressive disorders: an overview. In: Kleinman A, Good B, eds. Culture and Depression. Berkeley, CA: University of California Press; 1985:299-324.

48. Ro M. Moving forward: Addressing the health of Asian American and Pacific Islander women. Am J Public Health. 2002;92:516-9.

49. Carlson EB, Rosser-Hogan R. Mental health status of Cambodian refugees ten years after leaving their homes. Am J Orthopsychiatry. 1993;63:223-31.

50. Zhou HH, Koshakji RP, Silberstein DJ, et al. Racial differences in drug response: altered sensitivity to and clearance of propranolol in men of Chinese descent as compared to white Americans. N Engl J Med. 1989;320:565-70.

51. Zhou HH, Adedoyin A, Wilkinson GR. Differences in plasma binding of drugs between Caucasians and Chinese subjects. Clin Pharmacol Ther. 1990;48:10-7.

52. Davis A. Ethics and ethnicity: end-of-life decisions in four ethnic groups of cancer patients. Med Law. 1996;15:429-32.

53. Blackhall LJ, Murphy ST, Frank G, et al. Ethnicity and attitudes toward patient autonomy. JAMA. 1995;274:820-5.

54. Gold B, Socolar D. Report of the Boston Committee on Access to Health Care; 1987.

55. De La Cancela V, Chin JL, Jenkins YM. Community health psychology: empowerment for diverse communities. New York: Routledge; 1998.

56. Chin JL. Culturally competent health care. Public Health Rep. 2000;115:25-33.

6

Care of Arab Americans and American Muslims

MAYA M. HAMMOUD, MD

M. KAY SIBLANI, RN

Arab Americans and American Muslims are two separate and distinct population groups. The first is identified by ethnic origin, the second by religious affiliation. However, they share so many characteristics that, of necessity, they must be studied jointly. The similarities between the two groups arise from the fact that the Islamic faith sprang from and developed within an Arab society. Although its subsequent spread across the entire world has massively diversified the group of people who call themselves Muslim, the many Arab influences and components of the faith remain and are indeed embraced by non-Arab Muslims. Additionally, the profound impact that the practice of Islam has on an individual's everyday life necessarily renders all Muslim societies, whatever their cultural origin and even those with significant Christian minorities, comparable in significant ways, thus creating a worldwide "Muslim culture".

Major differences between American society and Arab/Muslim cultures have placed significant barriers to health care access for immigrants to the United States from the Arab and Muslim worlds. These barriers go far beyond simple language differences to encompass entire worldviews, concepts of health, illness, and recovery, and even the allocation of limited medical resources. Physicians are thus challenged in a number of ways when delivering care to these patients.

When groups of people in America identify themselves by their ethnicity, it is common for them to do so by hyphenating "American" to their ethnic origin—thus the term *Arab-American*. This inherently gives precedence to the American part of the identity, since "Arab" is simply an adjectival modifier. (The hyphen is nowadays often omitted.) When Muslims, on the other hand, identify themselves as American Muslims, they are considering their spiritual identity as primary and "American" as the modifier. This is not to detract from the importance of their American identity but to give precedence to spiritual matters over temporal ones. American Christians and Jews may do the same.

Nationality, Culture, and Religion

The Arab World consists of twenty-two countries or politically recognized states, most of them in the Middle East and northern Africa. In geographic terms, the Arab World includes Egypt, Tunisia, Libya, Algeria, Morocco, and Mauritania in northern Africa, as well as Lebanon, Syria, Jordan, and Palestine on the eastern border of the Mediterranean. The Arab World also encompasses the Persian or Arabian Gulf countries of Saudi Arabia, Yemen, Iraq, Kuwait, Oman, Bahrain, Qatar, and the United Arab Emirates. The east African island nation of Comores is included, as well as three interior African countries: Sudan, Somalia, and Djibouti.

The Arab World is a complex tapestry of politics, cultures, and religions. Over 200 million residents share the Arabic language as their mother tongue and are bound by a set of shared cultural values and worldview. Eighty percent of its residents are Muslims and twenty percent are Christian; however, Islam affects the culture of all residents. Their collective identification as Arab is a relatively new phenomenon, arising from political developments in the region in the past hundred years, and resurrecting a celebrated history that proceeded from the Arabian peninsula beginning in the 7th century with the advent of Islam.

There are some people from the Arab countries of the Middle East who share the culture and the language of the Arab World but prefer to identify themselves according to the particular sect of Christianity they follow rather than by the ethnic term *Arab*. Primary among them are the Assyrians and Chaldeans of Iraq, the Coptic Orthodox now found mostly in Egypt, and the Lebanese Maronite Catholics. They are all descendants of the earliest Christians but follow separate denominational divisions arising from theological differences over the nature of Christ and Papal supremacy, among other things (1). Although they all happen to be Christian rather than Muslim, that is not the single defining issue. There are many Christian Arabs who do strongly identify as Arabs. It is more for ancestral and political reasons that some Chaldeans from Iraq, for instance, prefer the term

Chaldean to *Arab,* or some Maronite Lebanese refer to their nationality as *Lebanese* but to their ethnicity as *Phoenician.*

Almost all available research and statistical data on this population use the term *Arab,* although *Middle Easterner* is sometimes used. The Middle East, however, does not consist of Arab countries exclusively; it also encompasses the Persian country of Iran and Turkey. Because the culture and faith of those living in the Middle East are so intertwined, however, cultural crossover between Arabs and the Muslim peoples of Iran and Turkey is common. In all of these Muslim countries, to varying degrees, Islamic guidelines and principles define everything from family law to acceptable public behavior.

The true anomaly among countries of the Middle East is, of course, the Jewish state of Israel. It is important to realize that to care competently for patients from Israel, one must look primarily to Jewish law and tradition for guidance.

There is a distinct Arab culture that defines the homelands of patients from the Arab World. Though Muslim and Christian Arabs have many values and practices in common, there are relevant issues specific to people of the Islamic faith. The Muslim World is a larger entity of which both the Arab World and the Middle East are subsets. In a secular society, it is easy to confuse ethnicity with religion when encountering people of other cultures whose faith is more evident than usual. We sometimes think everyone from India is Hindu and all Hindus are Indian, or that everyone from China is Buddhist and vice versa. In the case of Islam, an additional source of confusion is the fact that the religion was revealed to an Arab in what is now Saudi Arabia. Muslims believe the revelation came in the Arabic language, and that language has remained for over 1400 years a central part of the faith. Because of the many Arab influences on Muslim culture, many people think all Muslims are Arabs and that all Arabs are Muslim.

In truth, the term *Muslim* defines a broad category of people from many different ethnic and racial backgrounds. The Muslim World geographically refers collectively to those countries wherein the population is primarily of the Islamic faith. It includes all the countries of the Middle East except Israel, parts of Africa, and much of Asia; Indonesia, for instance, is the most populous Muslim nation on earth. Pakistan is a Muslim nation created by the 1948 division of India into separate Muslim and Hindu parts. Several of the former Soviet republics are Muslim states in which Muslim identity is only now becoming known since the breakup of the Soviet Empire. Many Americans believe in and/or practice the faith called Islam (see below). The world's Muslim population is estimated at close to a billion and a half, and Islam is considered to be the fastest growing religion in the world.

In summary, Arab patients are for the most part either Christian or Muslim; the majority of Arabs in the Middle East are Muslim, but many Arabs in the United States are Christian. Muslim patients may be Arab, but the majority of Muslims are not Arab, whether in America or in the world at large.

Immigration Patterns

Arabs have been immigrating to the United States in significant numbers since the late 1870s, when migrants from what are today Syria and Lebanon discovered the "entrepreneurial Eden" awaiting the industrious (2). These "Syrians" initiated the chain migration phenomenon that over the next 30 years brought more than 100,000 mostly Greek Orthodox immigrants to this country. In 1924, a stricter immigration law drastically reduced this influx.

Historians divide this period of "Syrian" immigration into two parts: from 1880 to 1910, which is called the "peddling" or "pioneer" period; and 1910 to 1930, called the "settled" period (2). Most of the pioneering immigrants were itinerant peddlers, known by their ubiquitous suitcases full of goods, suitcases that also symbolized their determination to return to their homeland one day. When confidence in the new country and a sense of permanence were established, gradually the suitcases gave way to retail establishments, more women immigrated, and the assimilation process became paramount. More than half of today's three million Arab Americans are third, fourth, and fifth generation descendants of these early pioneers.

Chaldeans began arriving in the Detroit area in the early 1900s. Their numbers remained relatively small until the 1960s. Those very early immigrants still spoke Aramaic, the language of their ancestors and of Jesus. Their linguistic and religious differences set them apart from the Arab World's majority. But persecution arising from political events in the Arab World has also been significant in setting them apart (3). Most Chaldeans today have lost the language of their ancestors and are proficient in Arabic and/or English instead.

The second wave of Arab immigration began after 1948 and intensified after 1967, partly in response to political events in the Middle East and partly due to the professional preferences clause of the Immigration and Naturalization Act of 1965. Compared with earlier immigrants, these new arrivals were better educated and more politicized. Most of them were Muslim. They were primarily from Egypt, Lebanon, Syria, Palestine, and Iraq. Chaldean immigration increased dramatically; the community saw a 600% growth rate in the 20 years from 1960-80.

Like later waves of immigrants from other parts of the world, these immigrants tended to cling to their cultural heritage and acculturate, rather than assimilate. This is an important distinction that implies retention of culture and acclimation to a new life rather than loss of native culture and disappearance into a new life.

Unlike the earliest waves of immigrants, the later immigrants have been subject to political, social, and economic upheaval in their homelands. By and large these immigrants have a deeper sense of being Arab rather than identifying as being from a particular country, and they are more vocal on issues relating to the world they left behind, especially as concerns United States foreign policy.

In contrast to Arab immigration, Muslim immigration did not become significant until after World War II. There is some fragmented evidence that Islam existed in the Americas even before Columbus, but certainly the first major immigration of Muslims to America was through the slave trade. Many slaves were taken from areas of Africa where Islam had already planted itself, such as the Senegambia region. No Islamic institutions were created by the enslaved Africans and their descendents; however, many tried to maintain an Islamic lifestyle. Most Muslim immigrants come from India and Pakistan and from the Arab World. The majority of the American Muslim population (42%), however, is African-American, blacks who have converted to the Muslim faith (4).

Demographics

Arab Americans

There are more than 3 million Arab Americans in the United States. Arab Americans are among the fastest growing ethnic populations in the major urban metropolitan centers of Detroit, Chicago, New York, and Los Angeles (5). As a group, Arab Americans are more highly educated than the average American but have a higher rate of poverty (5). The poverty rate among the more recent immigrants may be underestimated because of the wealth of the descendant group.

Lebanon, Iraq, Egypt, and Syria are the majority nations-of-origin. Six in ten Arabs are Syrian or Lebanese. It is unclear what percentage of Arab Americans is Muslim; recent estimates suggest that it may range from 10% to 30%. A disproportionately large number of medically underserved Arabs are Muslims.

Although Arab Americans can be found in all fifty states, there are strong concentrations in eleven: Michigan, California, New York, Massachusetts, Pennsylvania, Texas, Illinois, Ohio, New Jersey, Virginia, and Rhode Island. The most visible Arab American community is in metropolitan Detroit, where 350,000 Arab Americans reside; 50% are Muslim. This community also has the largest Chaldean population in the nation. Some states tend to have higher concentrations of Arabs from a particular country. Virginia's Arab American population has the highest percentage of Palestinians; New Jersey has the highest percentage of Egyptians; and there are more Arab Americans in Texas from the Arabian or Persian Gulf than in the other states (6).

Arab Americans as a whole are most likely to be found in the Northeast; however, Arab immigrants are more likely to be found in the West and Midwest. When compared with the general United States population, Arab Americans are twice as likely to be found in large urban areas than in rural ones. They are younger as a group than the general population and younger than most other ethnic groups. Arab Americans are more likely to be self-employed, less likely to work in government jobs, and much more likely to be in managerial and professional specialty occupations than the population at large. Arab Americans are more likely to be health professionals than the general population and other ethnic groups (7). Nearly half (46.5%) of all Arab Americans eighteen years and older speak a language other than English at home. This comparatively high percentage is testimony to the increasing numbers of second-wave immigrants. Only 10.4% of those 18 and older speak English not well or not at all (8).

This demographic overview reflects the entire Arab American community, including significant numbers of long assimilated members. The challenges presented to health care practitioners come from the group of recent immigrants, which has special needs that should be considered separately. The following summary of the Detroit-Dearborn community in Michigan, for instance, is taken from a health-needs assessment performed in 1998 by a local community center:

> The most recent figures indicate that more than 250,000 Arabs are living in the Detroit Metropolitan area, and it is estimated that about 27% of this population is below the poverty level standards, in comparison to roughly 5% of the general population. There are significant barriers to health care accessibility and acceptability for this community including language, lack of culturally competent and sensitive health services, transportation, financial security and inadequate knowledge related to health. The level of education of residents of the Arab community ranks lower than that of the general population ... the majority of community members are employed in the unskilled labor force and most of these jobs do not have health insurance benefits. It is estimated that 37% of the Arab American community lack health or medical insurance coverage, in comparison to the general population of Michigan where only 9% are uninsured. (9)

American Muslims

Because the Muslim community in America is so diverse, and because the one institution that ties all Muslims together, the mosque, is a relatively new phenomenon in this country, there are no extensive statistical data on American Muslims that can accurately reflect the community. The population has been estimated at 6 to 8 million, making it the second largest faith in the country, as well as the fastest growing. (Other estimates place the number lower; others as high as 10 million.) Its growth is due to a high conversion rate as well as increased immigration. The major Muslim groups in the United States break down as follows: African Americans, 42%; Indians and Pakistanis, 25%; and Arabs, 12% to 15%. The states with the highest Muslim populations are California, New York, New Jersey, Illinois, Indiana, and Michigan (4).

Overview of Islam

The religion of Islam prescribes a way of life that is relevant to health care delivery in the office, clinic, emergency room, in-patient ward, and community.

Whereas religion in the West tends to be regarded as a theological concept, in the East religion is a way of life, affecting everything from personal hygiene to socialization patterns. Again, where Americans tend to view themselves as human beings searching for spiritual experiences, Muslims are more likely to view themselves as spiritual beings having a human experience (10). The combined impact of an Eastern culture and an Eastern faith on the delivery of health care in a Western society can be profound (Case 6-1).

CASE 6-1   A 75-YEAR-OLD MALE ARAB MUSLIM WHO HAS PRAYERS INTERPRETED AS "STRANGE BEHAVIOR"

LB is a 75-year-old male Arab Muslim who speaks only a few words of English. He is admitted to the neurology floor with a stroke that causes him some confusion but appears to be improving quickly. At 6 A.M. a nurse finds him kneeling on the floor of his room raising his head up and down in what she considers a strange fashion and talking to himself. She is concerned that his behavior may be a sign of neurologic deterioration so she tries to get him back into bed. He resists her attempts and continues his activity. She tries again whereby he becomes extremely agitated and begins yelling at her in his own language. The frightened nurse leaves the room and calls security. When they arrive, the patient yells at them also. He is then forcibly placed into bed with four-point restraints.

When his son comes to the hospital later that day, the patient explains that he was trying to pray that morning but that the nurse kept interrupting him. The son angrily tells the staff that his father was praying and not acting abnormally. The nurse apologizes to the patient and his son.

DISCUSSION

This case illustrates the importance of a health care provider understanding the customs of other religions. Had the nurse been aware that Islamic prayer involves moving up and down while reciting verses from the *Qur'an*, this unfortunate and awkward episode would have been avoided.

Principles

Islam is one of the three major monotheistic religions in the world. It is classified as a religion, but it is actually a way of life, an all-encompassing set of rules for everyday living. For example, Muslims are commanded to join in community prayer on Fridays, and they do so at mosques. Western interpretation of this activity as Friday being the Muslim Sabbath is incorrect, however, because Muslims also are commanded to resume their daily activities right after the congregational prayer.

Muslims believe that God revealed His guidance for mankind in stages through the Major Prophets revered by Christians and Jews. Muslims hold Jesus as a major prophet whose words and deeds were God directed, but they do not regard him as the Son of God or the Savior of mankind. They do, however, believe in the Virgin Birth of Jesus, regarding it as a miracle from God. Arab Muslims believe they descended from Abraham's second son, Ishmael, and all Muslims believe Mohammed, born 600 years after Jesus, was another prophet—the last one—sent by God, the prophet who completed and perfected the message of the righteous way to live (11).

Practices

The Muslim religious institution is a *mosque;* religious leaders are called *imams.* Islam has five pillars of faith around which, to greater or lesser degrees depending on their level of observance, Muslims structure their lives (12). Because these five pillars are integral parts of a Muslim's everyday life, a health care giver is likely to encounter them with some regularity.

The first pillar of Islam is the *shahaadah,* or the proclamation of one's belief in the one and only God and in Mohammed's status as the last messenger of that God: "There is no God but God and Mohammed is the Messenger of God." This declaration of faith is said many times during prayer. It is also said at important times during the Muslim life cycle when health care providers are likely to be present.

The second pillar is *salat,* the obligatory performance of prayer five times every day following certain guidelines on form, content, and time. Prayers are said at dawn, noon, mid-afternoon, sunset, and nightfall. These prayers can be performed alone or communally, except the noon prayer on Friday, when men are required to perform communal prayer if possible.

(For discussion of prayer vis-à-vis the Islamic patient, see the section on Prayer below.)

The third pillar is payment of a religious tax called *zakat* (purification of one's money) that is partly to care for the needy in the community and partly to fulfill other objectives for the collective good. Two and one-half percent of one's earnings and assets are paid for distribution to the needy. Payment is calculated annually and is often made during Ramadan, the month of fasting.

The fourth pillar of Islam is fasting. Throughout the month of Ramadan, all Muslims fast from dawn until sunset, abstaining from food, drink, and sexual relations. (For discussion of fasting, see the section on Ramadan below.)

The fifth pillar of Islam is the pilgrimage to Makkah (Mecca) called the *Hadj*. It is enjoined upon every Muslim physically and financially able to make the trip once in his or her life. Muslims who make a communal pilgrimage are then conferred the title of *Hadj* for men and *Hadjah* for women.

The *Qur'an* is the Muslim Holy Book. The word *Qur'an* literally means "recitation" or "reading". Muslims believe Mohammed recited that which was revealed to him by God through the Angel Gabriel and that the recitation was memorized and set down in writing. The *Qur'an* in some ways corresponds to the Christian Bible, but while the Bible is recognized by most to be the work of many writers, Muslims believe the *Qur'an* consists entirely of the words of God as revealed to Mohammed (13).

The rules by which Muslims live are called *shari'ah,* or Islamic law, and are drawn primarily from the *Qur'an* and the *sunnah,* or the Prophet Muhammad's example. Everything a Muslim does can be placed into one of five categories of behavior:

- Obligatory (e.g., daily prayers)
- Recommended (e.g., getting married and raising a family)
- Permitted (e.g., shortened prayers while traveling)
- Allowed but not recommended (e.g., divorce)
- Absolutely forbidden (e.g., murder, adultery)

The application of *shari'ah* to new situations or scientific developments (organ donation, for example) is the concern of respected individuals or scholars called *'ulama.* They determine the Islamic position on these new events. Not surprisingly, however, there is often more than one Islamic opinion on many of the issues health care workers face with Muslim patients.

Impact of Culture on Health Care Delivery

Health Care and the Individual

Health care delivery in the United States is very much oriented toward the individual. Patient assessment, plans of care, and rules governing confidentiality are all based on a concept of individual rights that is unique to America. This policy of informed consent, however, may be at variance with the practices and beliefs of other cultures:

> Each element of informed consent, however, poses potential difficulties in US subcultures: full, truthful disclosure may be at variance with cultural beliefs about hope, wellness, and thriving of individuals. Autonomous decision-making may counter family-centered values and the social meanings of competency; and uncoerced choices may contradict cultural norms about, for example, obedience to the wishes of spouses or family elders. Physician conformance with variant cultural expectations may run afoul of informed consent requirements to make full and truthful disclosures and to allow autonomous decision-making (14).

Social and Family Structure

Three major social differences between the American and Arab/Islamic cultures significantly affect the delivery of health care: 1) the family system, 2) the importance of the individual versus the family and society, and 3) the assignment of primary gender roles.

Family System

The Arab/Islamic family system is residential or nonresidential extended as opposed to the nuclear or blended family system common in the United States. Health care providers must deal with the Arab/Muslim *family*, not just the Arab/Muslim *patient*. A strong family unit is the cornerstone of Arab/Muslim life. Care of, and obedience to, one's parents are important. Elders are respected for their age and wisdom and are often consulted on matters relevant to health care. Children usually do not leave home until they marry. Relatives from overseas often become members of the household after immigration. Parents and aged relatives are almost always kept at home when they become infirm.

The Arab/Muslim patient tends to have more interaction with his or her family and community than does the average American patient. The term *next of kin* may have no meaning to an Arab family (15).

Individual versus Family and Society

The needs of the Arab/Muslim individual are secondary to the benefit of the larger social structures: first the family, then society at large. The idea of having one's own life to live regardless of what the family may want or what society may find acceptable does not exist in traditional Arab/Muslim society. Arabs believe loyalty to one's family and the benefit of one's actions to society must take precedence over personal wants and desires. Arab patients are likely to define themselves and their individual worth as relative to, rather than independent of, the rest of their family. Major decisions usually involve all members of the extended family, especially the men. Full disclosure and patient autonomy may even be nonexistent. Two examples may be given:

1. Married immigrant women who are illiterate in English and unprepared to deal with complex medical issues may expect and prefer that health care workers deal with their husbands, and usually away from the bedside. This approach may raise questions of liability as well as ethical dilemmas for providers. Usually these issues can be resolved by documenting in the medical record the reason for deviating from usual practice. If a woman prefers not to be included in discussions about her care, the provider should ask the patient if it is acceptable to discuss her case with her husband outside her presence. The provider then documents the woman's permission and any ensuing conversations with the husband.

2. In the Arab culture, telling a patient that he or she is terminally ill is sometimes not acceptable. Arabs feel that disclosing terminal status to a patient accomplishes nothing except the taking away of hope; and, in spite of what medical science indicates, only God knows when someone is going to die. The family believes it is their role to protect the patient and to deal with the

issues of a terminal illness or serious diagnosis. This cultural norm may preclude full disclosure to the patient. However, this preference is not universal among Muslims of other ethnicities. Many Muslims will deal very straightforwardly with terminal diagnoses and impending death.

Among Arabs, discussions about diagnosis, prognosis, and treatment options are likely to be undertaken *with* the family. This is an area that requires careful thought and documentation to meet the needs of both the patient and the system in which he or she is receiving care. Independent ethical review may be indicated to explore the most appropriate way of handling certain situations. The respect for human dignity upon which the doctrine of informed consent is based also dictates that health care providers obtain consent in ways that are comprehensible and consistent with the patient's language, customs, and culture. The fact that individuals give deference to the views of family and community, and even prefer therapeutic discourse to occur with family members, does not negate the need for individual assent to medical treatment (14).

Gender Roles

Islam assigns separate primary life roles for men and for women. Men are the primary breadwinners, and women are primarily responsible for the raising of children. Note that these are *primary* roles, not *exclusive* roles. In some Arab communities, if a woman can manage the care of her home and children adequately, she is encouraged to seek knowledge and is free to have a career. Arab society, however, is strictly patriarchal and the men in the family, at least publicly, make final decisions. The section on Gender Roles and Segregation below provides a fuller discussion of this topic.

Concepts of Health, Illness, and Recovery

Different cultures have different concepts of health and illness. Muslims may see illness as a test of both their faith in God and their patience in a time of distress. For example, hospice nurses often have a hard time dealing with a Muslim's perception of terminal illness, since they have spent years learning to help patients live with impending death. In this situation, they may have to recognize that what they consider denial of reality, the patient may see as a strengthening of his or her faith. What is important is to meet the patient's needs in whatever context the patient is comfortable, rather than to pull out a monolithic plan of care and expect the patient to follow it regardless.

Belief in the "evil eye" is not uncommon outside the United States. Many cultures (e.g., in southern Europe and the Middle East) believe that envy of something owned by another person causes the "evil eye" to be cast on that person. If the person becomes ill, it is because of this curse. When patients have these beliefs, it is important to acknowledge their existence and the validity the patient gives them. Dispelling these beliefs should not be a goal. Instead, one should focus on the fact that whatever the cause of the problem, the treatment and the chances for recovery are the same (Case 6-2).

In Arab culture, total abdication of responsibility from one's usual activities is believed to be necessary for full recovery from illness. This belief creates a dependency that interferes with the usual approach to recovery in

---

CASE 6-2   A MUSLIM WOMAN WHO BELIEVES HER NIPPLE INFECTION IS CAUSED BY THE "EVIL EYE"

A physician in a large urban hospital is concerned about a new mother who has been admitted three times in six weeks with a post-partum nipple infection. The mother, a practicing Muslim, firmly believes the infection is caused by the "evil eye" cast by a neighbor envious of her new baby. The practitioner does not know how to address the situation.

Upon consultation with several individuals learned in Muslim culture, the practitioner is advised not to try to disabuse the patient of her belief in the "evil eye". She is to tell the patient, however, that there are other causes of nipple infection and she is to provide treatment and prevention strategies. Consequently, the patient is advised to combine the practitioner's recommended treatment with her own approaches to dealing with the problem.

DISCUSSION

This case illustrates the importance of understanding a patient's explanatory model of illness and the need to negotiate treatment strategies when the doctor's and patient's views of illness differ.

the United States (i.e., attempting early activity and progressive resumption of one's normal life). Patients with this belief may require teaching and/or extensive family involvement before making progress in work-focused rehabilitation. In dealing with these challenges, effective strategies include adjusting one's own expectations, using culturally competent "consultants" from the community, and educating the entire family about the importance of appropriately paced rehabilitation. Rehabilitation staff, for instance, may have to focus on teaching family members how to care for the patient, rather than emphasizing steps the patient must take to attain full recovery as soon as possible.

Communication and Language

In many instances, characteristic responses to particular messages may be diametrically opposed in the Arab and traditional American cultures. The results range from confusion at best to outright harm in the worst situations. As with other ethnic communities of recent origin, immigrant Arabs and Muslims may not possess facility with the English language. Interpreters are especially needed for older patients who are new immigrants or who have never learned English. (Younger patients tend to have learned to speak English before immigrating.) This obvious communication barrier can have profound impact on every aspect of a patient's medical course. Interpreters must be carefully chosen and monitored. Using first-generation children as interpreters can have adverse consequences on important family power structures and patient self-esteem. Family and friends may omit important parts of the conversation without informing the practitioner. Those not proficient in English may relay inaccurate information. Competent medical interpreters are proficient in both English and Arabic and understand medical terminology and the Arab culture (Case 6-3) (16).

Arabs use their language in a different manner than Americans. Whereas Americans use language primarily to communicate an idea, Arabs use language as a sort of social lubricant. Their communication style is highly contextual, meaning that one must take into account the context of the speech as well as the words that are actually spoken. The words may be modified to save face, to make everyone present comfortable, or to preserve social etiquette on a particular occasion. The listener is expected to pick up on nonverbal cues and to use common sense, relationship history, and other factors in interpreting the meaning of what is being said (17).

CASE 6-3   A 33-YEAR-OLD SAUDI ARABIAN WOMAN WHO SPEAKS NO ENGLISH AND IS TERMINALLY ILL

MS is a 33-year-old woman from Saudi Arabia who presents to the emergency room with an acute abdomen. She does not speak English and her husband, who acts as interpreter, speaks English poorly. She is taken to the operating room and found to have extensive pelvic infection, which necessitates a hysterectomy and removal of both ovaries. The patient is then hospitalized in the intensive care unit for several weeks due to severe sepsis. She continues to have multiple problems with fistulas, however, and undergoes a bowel resection. Final pathology demonstrates metastatic colon cancer. Again, because no interpreter is available, the physician must explain her situation as best he can to the husband.

The patient is seen in clinic for follow-up by an Arabic-speaking physician who realizes that she does not understand the extent of her disease. She is unaware that her cancer is metastatic. The physician arranges a meeting with the patient and her family to discuss her condition. When she learns about her poor prognosis, the patient arranges for her three young children to fly to the United States from Saudi Arabia.

DISCUSSION

This case illustrates how language barriers affect care. Because the patient did not speak English and her husband understood it imperfectly, she did not receive appropriate information about her disease and prognosis. To deliver the best possible care when patients do not speak English, it is important to have a trained interpreter to communicate with the patient and family. Relying on a family member who cannot speak English well can lead to miscommunication and a false understanding of the medical situation.

Arabs believe that words have a power of their own: that saying something may help make it come true. Consequently they make extensive use of euphemisms and are reluctant to speak directly about negative issues or outcomes (e.g., the phrase "a little sick" may be used for someone who is, in fact, very ill).

Other differences in language use are important to the physician. For example, to the question "How are you?" Muslims will invariably answer the equivalent of "Thank God I am as good as I am" (*alhamdullilah*). Most Arabs tend to repeat this response until they are comfortable in a given situation (e.g., a relationship of trust with the physician). Questioning using different phrasing may then reveal information not initially evident that may be helpful in performing health care needs assessment. It is also helpful to avoid the use of the first person when discussing issues of a negative nature. For instance, when talking about the risks of a particular surgery, a physician should say "A patient in this situation might experience a wound infection" rather than "You may experience. . . ."

Arab speech is often repetitive and flowery as opposed to short and simple, a consequence of the Arabic language having a coordinated-type structure rather than the subordinate structure of English narrative. This characteristic often carries over into Arab use of the English language. Thus it is important to take time for the social courtesies. Haste is often mistaken for rudeness and can get the patient-physician relationship off to a rocky start. An entire family's sense of honor can hinge on a show of public respect.

It is considered impolite in Arab culture to say "no" to another person. Whereas an American may respond "no" to the question "Do you understand?" and not consider it in any way rude, an Arab might answer "yes" out of a desire not to be impertinent or disrespectful. Thus it is important for the health care provider to try to avoid "yes, no" questions. Ask for concrete information instead. By the same token, when having to give a negative response to a patient request, try to avoid answering with a simple 'no' but rather elaborate and soften your reply. Incidentally, the Arab way of indicating "no" nonverbally looks like the American nod of the head for "yes", often accompanied by a clicking of the tongue.

Time

Arabs view time as their slave. They are not as clock-conscious as Americans, and many show up late for appointments. This is an ongoing problem for health care institutions and doctors' offices. However, it is important for the practitioner to realize that tardiness does not exhibit a lack of respect for the appointment or the person. Respect and promptness are not linked.

Self-Esteem

In the Arab culture one's sense of honor comes from family name and ancestral lineage. It is important to realize that whatever one says or does to a person of Arab heritage is said or done to the entire extended family. Conversely, whatever an Arab says or does is as if said or done by everyone in his or her family. Arabs grow up hearing the word *ayb* ("shame, shameful") on a frequent basis. They are taught "This is *ayb*" and "That is *ayb*," and they are expected to govern themselves in such a way that they do not bring shame upon their family. The honor of the family name is paramount. Sharing personal information is thus much less easily done in Arab culture.

Mental illness and depression may be considered not only culturally taboo but religiously taboo as well. Many Muslims feel one cannot be depressed if one is following the tenets of the faith, and they may not acknowledge the legitimacy of anti-depressants. When dealing with adolescents and the various crises they face, the practitioner must remain aware of the need to maintain family honor and traditional parental authority while remaining cognizant of the needs and rights of the adolescent.

Mistrust of Institutions

Generally speaking, Arab culture is based upon personal relationships, whereas Americans are used to dealing with institutions (18). Americans may not trust certain individuals in an institution but trust the institution as a whole. Arabs, on the other hand, may not trust the institution as a whole but trust certain individuals within it. Thus one bad experience with a staff member can damage an Arab patient's experience with a health care organization; one good experience can make up for a number of institutional blunders.

Because they are not accustomed to concerning themselves with the protocols of a medical institution, Arabs may expect providers and others to make exceptions in order to meet their personal needs (see the section on Time above). Understanding the cultural ethos behind this behavior can render an otherwise judgment-laden interpretation of this expectation more neutral and permit a more effective response to it (Case 6-4).

CASE 6-4   ARAB PATIENTS WHO ARE UNHAPPY WITH AVAILABLE APPOINTMENTS

A scheduling receptionist at a major university medical center is frustrated because Arab patients needing physical therapy are never happy with the available appointments and always want to investigate other possibilities. Often there is no apparent reason for patient discontent with the available dates and times.

DISCUSSION

Arab patients tend not to believe that a receptionist automatically offers the best possible appointment. This belief may arise from distrust of institutions and a feeling that personal needs are more important than those of the institution. Roots in a bargaining culture, where it is normal to negotiate for the best possible price or arrangement, may be important as well. The strategies most likely to assist the receptionist in dealing effectively with these patients and their families are 1) understanding the reasons behind their behavior, 2) listening to their personal concerns, and 3) ensuring they have the opportunity to negotiate an agreeable appointment time. For example, rather than the receptionist telling the patient that several appointments are available, a mutually agreed upon appointment time should be negotiated between the two parties.

Establishing personal relationships is important when planning or delivering care. Because they have complex relationships with extended families, Arab patients may not have the same ideas as many Americans about forming therapeutic relationships with health care workers. They may not want care, they may just want cure. Patients may get their emotional support elsewhere. Relations with health care personnel other than the physician may be more social than therapeutic (19).

Often, immigrant Arabs face communication barriers, financial difficulties, loss of self-esteem, intergenerational conflict, and government actions and politics that dictate the way in which they respond to providers in the health care setting. In many immigrant communities, people who have obtained high levels of education in their native lands hold low-level positions at minimum wage due to differences in licensing or immigration work rules. This often creates high levels of stress, which can affect health outcomes and increase health-related financial expenditures (20,21).

Arab immigrants come from many countries where there is mistrust in the government that runs many of the hospitals. They are likely to view some interventions of the health care system as more related to the secret police than to the Hippocratic oath. When providers ask detailed personal questions or request information about the home (in preparation for home care, for example), patients may become suspicious of the motives. It is important to explain why the information is necessary and how it is relevant to care.

Impact of Faith on Health Care Delivery

Perhaps the best way to begin this section is to note that Islam is a very flexible religion. The maintenance of health and life is of paramount concern, and whatever is necessary toward that end is acceptable. A famous verse from the *Qur'an* states that if pork were the only food available to prevent a Muslim from starving, it would be incumbent upon him or her to eat the pork (22).

While Islam is flexible, Muslims may not be. In general, anything that is necessary to save a life and for which there is no available alternative is religiously acceptable. At times, the health care practitioner may have to go to the trouble of providing alternatives not readily available. At other times, Muslim patients may need directives to understand the need for something not usually tolerated.

There is no one monolithic Islamic doctrine to which to turn for the solution to every dilemma. For example, recently a hospital with many Arab patients from the same small sect of Islam consulted with two religious leaders overseas on the legality of discontinuing life support on a particular patient. The two gave opposing decisions.

Culture versus Religion

Adding to this complexity is a phenomenon borne of the close interaction between culture and faith in Islam. Many Muslims spend their entire lives believing some cultural directives to be religious in origin, because their faith does direct so much of their daily lives. The widespread Arab cultural practice of male circumcision is not commanded by the *Qur'an,* however, and the practice of female circumcision is religiously unacceptable. Muslim patients may require education to assist them in determining whether a particular health care directive actually compromises their Islamic faith. Individuals and organizations in the community can serve as resources to help resolve conflicts. In an emergency, a Muslim colleague can be invaluable, if only to provide comfort to a patient or family, though certainly not all Muslim health care providers are experts on matters related to Islam. Professional consultation is required to educate and prepare a staff to deal with Muslim patients on a regular basis.

A major example of confusion between culture and religion concerns fatalism. Despite the reputation Islam suffers for being fatalistic, Muslims educated in the faith know that fatalism is the antithesis of Islam. The consequences of this fatalistic attitude on health are noncompliance (neglecting or refusing treatment) and lack of recognition of the importance of lifestyle changes to improve health. Anecdotal evidence in the Dearborn Muslim community, for instance, suggests a higher rate of smoking and less awareness of its adverse consequences among new immigrants. Education and acculturation influence the degree to which this attitude exists.

Gender Roles and Segregation

Much of the gender differentiation that exists in Arab culture arises from Islam. There are wide variations in the role and social position of women in Muslim communities. Islam permeates all of society; even Christian Arab women are affected by its dictates, although not as strictly. Gender differences and the subject of sexuality are openly dealt with in the *Qur'an.* In the interest of a moral social order, Islamic teachings aim to ensure the protection and privacy of women as well as their rights.

It is difficult to generalize on this issue as far as practice. There are Muslim women who are physicians and attorneys and professors, all with full careers as well as families and active social lives. Others rarely leave their homes, speak little English, and do not appear when their husbands are entertaining. This variation is owing to several factors: culture, level of education, origin of the family (rural or urban), among others. Some segregation of the sexes exists in most communities, and protecting women's modesty is a universal concern among Muslims.

Both culture and religious practices affect the degree of segregation. Women may be separated from men in the prayer room of a mosque, but not in other sections of the mosque, at other events in the mosque, or socially outside the mosque. More commonly, women and men are seated in separate sections during lectures or dinners at the mosque and during social events as well. The separation is not seen as offensive or discriminatory by most observant Muslim women, although there is no doubt that controversy does exist over the practice. Often, however, women who are part of the Muslim community by birth but not necessarily observant generate this controversy. The vociferousness of the complaint often is directly related to the degree of the practice.

Hospital and office personnel must respect a woman's modesty during medical and nursing care in order to avoid offending or frightening her. Sometimes a Muslim woman will refuse bed baths during a hospital stay because of her fear of immodesty. A Muslim woman will not tolerate careless exposure of her body and will avoid any bed bath that might be interrupted by a group of physicians, including males, gathering round the bed with the patient barely covered. *Observant Muslim women are inculcated with the idea of modesty and chastity throughout their lives.* This is perhaps the single most important point for physicians to keep in mind when caring for Muslim women.

Except in emergency situations a Muslim woman will usually not accept care from a male caregiver if it involves uncovering her body or being alone with the caregiver. Some families are very strict about this. In general, the reverse is also true: Muslim men will not accept care from an unrelated female caregiver. Muslims may not even want an interpreter or translator of the opposite sex.

Some Muslims will not shake the hand of a person of the opposite sex. A Muslim man who will not shake the hand of a woman will sometimes place his right hand on his chest and bow slightly to acknowledge the introduction. Others may not have the social skill to do this. It is best for caregivers of both sexes not to offer their hands to the opposite sex unless invited to do so. Direct eye contact with the opposite sex may also be avoided by some Muslims. This combination of no handshaking and no eye contact can be very disconcerting and is often misinterpreted, especially by Western women. While the Arab men are according these women their highest respect, the latter often feel ignored or treated as less than equal. Finally, direct physical contact is often used as a comforting measure in the health care field. It is not unusual to hold hands, pat the arm, or give a hug at times of stress, pain, or grief. These gestures may be deemed inappropriate between a man and a woman, however, and can alienate Muslim patients rather than comfort them.

If cross-gender care is imperative, in emergency or teaching situations, for instance, it is considered acceptable. The use of gloves to prevent direct skin contact can sometimes make the situation more tolerable.

Female Dress

Almost always, what a Muslim woman wears is the cultural interpretation of "Islamic" dress, and such dress varies widely. A common aspect is the covering of the head. Veiling was done in pre-Islamic times and originated as a form of class distinction. It was not confined to Arabia. The women of the higher classes wore veils to distinguish themselves and to hide themselves from the view of other men. Veiling is different from covering the head. Many Muslim women wear Western clothes but "scarf" or "cover", as they call it. The head cover is worn in the house if anyone other than immediate and near family males is present and at all times outside the home. Some women only cover in the mosque or at Muslim gatherings. An observant woman who covers will keep her scarf on while an inpatient. There is no religious significance to the scarf itself. A nurse or doctor may to ask the patient to remove it when necessary to provide medical or nursing care. Female patients may post a sign outside their hospital rooms requesting that men knock before entering so they can adjust their covering.

It is important to understand that Muslim women who cover usually do so because they want to. They view the *hidjab* as an empowering tool. They appreciate the privacy and respect covering accords them. Some also believe that, in a work setting, covering takes the emphasis off the way they look and places it on their performance, giving them greater equality with men. Perhaps one of the greatest advantages to covering is that it identifies a woman as a practicing Muslim, thus leaving no doubt about what kind of behavior she will accept from others and the behavior others can expect from her.

Cleanliness and Personal Hygiene

The concepts of *taharah* (Islamically clean) and *nadjasah* (not Islamically clean) govern every Muslim's life to a great extent because one must be in a state of *taharah* to pray. Once the cleansing ritual is performed, the person remains in a state of purity fit for prayer. Falling asleep, passing stool, urine, or gas, vomiting, discharging blood or pus from any part of the body, or losing reasoning ability due to drugs or intoxicants breaks the state of purity. A complete bath is required before prayer, after sexual intercourse, after wet dreams, and after the end of a woman's period or confinement from childbirth, not to exceed 10 and 40 days, respectively.

Running water while bathing is very important historically. Sitting or lying in a tub of water without first washing and rinsing and draining the soiled water is unacceptable to many Muslims. In the hospital patients may object to basin or tub baths on this principle, or they may demand that the nurse or assistant frequently change the water. Showering is generally preferred and should not present problems unless showering compromises a woman's modesty. Muslim patients may not be comfortable with the use of toilet paper only, believing that cleansing with water is also necessary. Muslims need assurance that items shared with other patients (e.g., blood pressure cuffs, bedside commodes, geriatric chairs) are cleaned before use and may insist on observing the cleaning.

Prayer

As mentioned earlier, prayer is one of the five pillars of Islam. Muslims generally desire privacy while praying. Do not walk in front of a person who is praying or interrupt him or her, because prayers must be performed again if concentration is not maintained. In Islam, those who are able to perform the physical components of prayer are commanded to do so, but those who cannot must pray sitting or lying down. Patients may also want their beds to be positioned facing Makkah (i.e., they wish to face the Holy City when they sit up). Women who have their period or who have just given birth may not pray. Hospitals with large Muslim populations may want to provide a place for public prayer.

Halaal and *Haraam*

The daily life of the strictly observant Muslim is governed by the concepts of *halaal* and *haraam*. *Halaal* comprises behaviors considered acceptable by Islamic law. Unacceptable behaviors are *haraam*, which includes prohibitions against pork, alcohol and intoxicating drugs, extramarital sex, gambling, and usury (23); some patients may reject organ donation on the basis of *haraam*.

Halaal contains dietary rules similar to the kosher rules of the Jewish faith. Animals, including poultry, must be slaughtered in a ritualistic manner that drains the blood from the animal while the name of God is invoked. Some Muslims do not insist on *halaal* food, whereas other hospitalized patients may request food from home to ensure that is *halaal.* Vegetarian meals suffice if *halaal* food is not available.

In general, medical or survival needs exempt one from *halaal* laws, although some Muslims will avoid alcohol in over-the-counter medications. Rarely, some Muslims may object to the use of alcohol on the skin as an antiseptic. It may be necessary to reassure patients about the use of narcotics when they are necessary.

Ramadan

Because Ramadan is the month during which Mohammed received his revelations from God through the Angel Gabriel, it is considered holy. Fasting from dawn to sunset during Ramadan is required by every Muslim in good health who is not traveling. Muslims are exempted from fasting by the *Qur'an* if they are ill or their health is threatened. Women do not fast while menstruating, but they must make up those days at another time in the year before next Ramadan. During pregnancy or nursing, fasting is dictated by medical concerns.

Fasting involves abstaining from drinking, eating, and smoking, and refraining from sexual relations. Specific rules covering the fast concern everything from taking medicine to brushing teeth. Intravenous fluids or injections, total parenteral nutrition, intramuscular injections, and blood or blood component transfusions invalidate a fast; however, patients who require these interventions generally are too ill to fast (Case 6-5).

Muslims receive much spiritual comfort from the fast. Therefore hospital patients may want to fast even though their illness exempts them from this requirement. If patients can safely fast from dawn to sunset, taking their nourishment during other hours, fasting may assist recovery.

Specific Health Care Issues

Women's Health Issues

Female circumcision is not an Islamic rule but a culturally practiced tradition, one gradually being eradicated. Temporary birth control is acceptable

---

CASE 6-5   A PREGNANT MUSLIM WHOSE FASTING IS HARMFUL TO HER HEALTH

BN is a 23-year-old Muslim woman who has been receiving prenatal care at a university clinic. She is at 28 weeks' gestation when Ramadan begins. During a routine office visit, she reports that she has suffered many episodes of dizziness and has passed out twice since she began fasting a few days earlier. The physician advises her to stop fasting because of the deleterious effect on her and her baby's health. The patient insists that she continue fasting as required by her religion. A few days later she is admitted to the hospital for dehydration and pre-term contractions.

Her physician consults a Muslim religious leader who explains that Muslims are exempted from fasting if their health is threatened, as stated in the Qur'an. The physician discusses the consultation with the patient, quoting the appropriate reference. The patient is satisfied and stops fasting. She delivers a healthy baby 2 months later.

DISCUSSION

This case illustrates how understanding the religious beliefs of a patient and consulting an expert can help resolve a doctor-patient dilemma.

---

in Islam, although some Muslims make a distinction between pre- and post-conception methods. Birth control pills are an example of an acceptable pre-conception method because there is no aborting of a fertilized egg. Tubal ligation and vasectomy may be considered unacceptable because they are permanent. The morning-after pill and the IUD for emergency contraception are examples of post-conception birth control methods that some Muslims do not find acceptable. Assisted reproductive techniques or the use of fertility drugs and procedures to enable pregnancy are allowed if they do not violate the sanctity of the marital relationship or raise questions about a child's parentage.

Vaginal exams of unmarried girls may present a problem because virginity is important in Arab culture and in Islam. A pelvic examination in a woman who has not been sexually active should be avoided if possible (Case 6-6). Rectal and breast examinations are acceptable. Muslim girls and women are generally more comfortable with a female physician. If one is not available, a female chaperone or family member should be present when the patient is examined.

CASE 6-6   A 24-YEAR-OLD EGYPTIAN WOMAN WHO REFUSES A PELVIC EXAMINATION ON RELIGIOUS AND MORAL GROUNDS

SL is a 24-year-old single woman from Egypt with end-stage renal disease who comes to the United States for evaluation for kidney transplant. She needs a full physical examination including a pelvic exam and Pap smear. The patient declines the pelvic exam because she has never been sexually active and fears never being able to marry if she "loses her virginity". An Arab Muslim physician speaks with the patient and her family about performing the exam without disrupting the hymenal ring but to no avail. The patient misses several appointments at the gynecology clinic and continues to decline physically.

A compromise acceptable to both parties is finally reached. The patient qualifies for the kidney transplant after undergoing an external pelvic exam and pelvic ultrasonography.

DISCUSSION

Despite providing appropriate counseling from a culturally and religiously sensitive physician, this patient continued to refuse a pelvic exam even though her condition was life threatening. It is often possible, however, to reach a compromise between medical necessities and a patient's moral and religious beliefs. Though Pap smear guidelines recommend the procedure in women starting at the age of 18, a woman who has never had intercourse is at extremely low risk for cervical cancer because most cervical cancers are associated with sexually transmitted infections.

Medicine and Surgery

Intravenous therapy and transfusion of blood and blood products are acceptable in Islam, as is the donation of blood. Less well-educated Muslim patients may believe otherwise and may need counseling from someone they respect as knowledgeable about Islam. Medicine or other products made from pork (e.g., pork insulin and heparin) are unacceptable unless no other options are available.

Arabs and Muslims do not typically discuss sexually transmitted infections (STI). The prohibition of extramarital sex theoretically precludes a public health problem with STI. In practice however, especially in America, many men and women do not necessarily follow the cultural and religious recommendations. Physicians should screen Arabs and Muslims for risky sexual behavior and provide education about STI. However, many patients will find questioning on this subject offensive.

Mental Health and Substance Abuse

Muslim physicians, preceding the work of Jung and Freud, founded many concepts of mental illness. On a cultural level, however, the idea of mental illness may not be well accepted. It is often helpful to frame descriptions of mental illness in pathophysiological terms (e.g., describing depression as a chemical imbalance in the brain) rather than as a psychological process. In many cultures, mental illness is a source of shame, and careful and discreet family counseling is important to the prognosis of the patient.

Substance abuse occurs in this population as in any other. However, unlike those Americans who publicly admit to a drug problem and seeking treatment for it, Arabs and Muslims are reluctant to openly acknowledge such a problem. For Arab Americans whose ethnic identity and cultural mores are more integral to their lives than Islam, providing treatment outside the community and culture may be best. Conversely, Muslims whose Islamic identity is paramount may require care from Muslim institutions and caregivers with skills related to treating mental health problems, so that Islamic dictates are followed.

Death and Dying

Religious issues become important when death is imminent. Muslims believe that the present life is only a trial preparation for the next realm of existence and that a just God would not create man and be unconcerned about his ultimate fate. Basic articles of faith include an afterlife, a Day of Judgment, resurrection, and heaven and hell.

Death is part of the Muslim life cycle and is regarded as such. Physicians should support patients in carrying out their usual activities even when they have a serious illness. There is an obligation, however, to do everything possible to promote life and restore health. In Islam, death is defined as total departure of the soul from the body. Chemotherapy, radiation therapy, and medically indicated experimental drugs do not present a problem and are usually accepted by the observant Muslim and the Arab patient. Assisted suicide is unacceptable to the observant Muslim. Arabs are often very vocal and very physical in their grieving. It is a good idea to provide a place where a large family can gather with some privacy, with the body if possible, to facilitate the grieving process.

Muslim customs surrounding death are based on the belief that one's body belongs to God. Muslim custom requires a total body wash of the body at the time of death. Muslims avoid autopsies, embalming, and cosmetic reconstruction if possible, following the Prophet's tradition of simply returning the body to the earth from which it came. Some believe, however, that autopsies are allowable if there is an urgent need to learn the cause of death, in the interest of science, or in the interest of saving someone from blame in the death. Embalming is generally done only if the body is being flown overseas for burial. Cremation is not accepted. If an autopsy is important, consultation and guidance from a religious leader may be helpful to the family.

Advance Directives

Many Arab and Muslim patients, particularly immigrants and less educated people, will be culturally and religiously unprepared for the use of Advance Directives. One cultural barrier comes from the Arab custom of assigning power to words. Many Arabs may feel that talking about end-of-life scenarios invites disaster. Unless the purpose and use of an Advance Directive is clearly understood, many Muslims may perceive its use as an indication that a physician knows when a person is going to die, knowledge only God possesses.

Presenting Advance Directives at the time of admission can be traumatizing for patients and families who have never heard of the concept. They may believe that the hospital staff know something they are not sharing or that the patient's condition is far more serious than revealed. Either discuss

Advance Directives before admission or delay discussion until the patient and family have been oriented to the hospital and clinical situation.

Advance Directives can be very helpful to Arabs and Muslims if they understand their purpose: to prevent the artificial prolonging of the dying process. One way to help families understand is to explain that if the patient cannot sustain his or her own life and the physician believes medical intervention will not change the outcome, then, at certain times, keeping a patient on life-support or performing CPR might be attempting to interfere with the will of God.

Code Status/Life Support

The issues of code status and life support with critically ill patients are not easier to handle or less complex in the Arab/Muslim population than in the general population. Every situation requires personalized attention, but the following general guidelines may be considered helpful:

1. Muslims are as concerned with spiritual death as they are with physical death. Both must occur before death is considered final.
2. Arab/Muslim families experience the same diversity of opinions of treatment of the critically ill as the general population. Withholding nutrition and fluids is generally unacceptable in Islam, however.
3. In general, Arab/Muslim patients will follow the advice of their physician as to whether a patient should be placed on life support. They have the highest respect for physicians and feel that they have the knowledge and training to best make such decisions. Once a patient is on life support, however, it is generally extremely difficult for a Muslim family to agree to discontinue it.

Muslims may not accept brain death as evidence of death, even when the brain stem is involved. One Islamic ruling outlines three possible outcomes for a patient on life support:

1. The patient begins to breath on his own, his heart beats normally, and life support is removed as soon as the patient is no longer in danger.
2. The heart no longer beats nor is there spontaneous breathing even with life support. In this situation, life support is removed because there is no doubt that death has occurred.

3. The third possibility is the one that causes dilemmas in intensive care units. The patient is brain dead but under life support, his heart beats, and there may be spontaneous breathing. If the doctor feels the patient will die after life support is removed, then it is permissible to remove it. Death should not be pronounced until all signs of life are gone. If there is a possibility the patient may live after removal of life support, then it is not permissible to remove it until death occurs or the patient no longer needs it (24).

It is difficult to convince loved ones that death has occurred when they see indications of life in the patient. Explaining brain death to Arab/Muslim families as a "serious sign of impending death" may help them make the decision to remove life support.

Organ Transplants

Donation and receipt of organs for transplant from a living donor are usually acceptable as long as the donor's life is not threatened and the donation is not part of the external body (e.g., an eye). Whether organs are to be donated or received after death remains a controversial issue and should be handled on an individual basis. Some Arabs/Muslims believe that because the act of donation serves humanity, it is acceptable and commendable. Others believe that organ donation from someone who has died violates the body.

Arab/Muslim families generally require that an individual give permission for organ donation and will not consent as next of kin. It is important to work closely with the family about when to take an organ, because Muslims believe the soul is still present if there are any signs of life. Thus an effort to procure a donor upon declaration of brain death but before life support is removed can be counter-productive. A religious ruling can be found to support various opinions on organ donation.

Conclusion

Patients from the Arab World and others of the Islamic faith present significant challenges to the health care practitioner, which if unmet can result in less than optimal care. For both ethical and financial reasons, it is incumbent upon the health system to provide culturally competent care. Ethically, physicians are mandated to interact with patients in ways that are helpful and healing. Financially, excessive lengths of stay, readmissions, lack of appropriate lifestyle changes, noncompliance, and lack of preventive screening all feed into higher health care costs.

In the cost-conscious health care environment we function in today, many administrators are reluctant to allocate funds for education and cultural programs. Knowing the impact that culture and faith have on the delivery of health care to Arab-Americans and American Muslims, we should work toward achieving health care intervention that is culturally congruent. As the patient population becomes ever more diverse, the need for culturally appropriate health care delivery becomes ever more important.

Summary of Communication Issues in Caring for Arab Americans and American Muslims

- Tradition of using euphemisms (e.g., "a little sick" may actually mean "very ill")
- Unwillingness to talk about negative outcomes because of fear that talking about them might make them come true
- Reluctant to disclose personal information; may need to be asked a question more than once (e.g., "How do you feel?") before feeling comfortable enough to give a medically accurate answer
- For patients with limited or no English, an interpreter is necessary; be careful using family members or friends of the patient because they may omit important information or translate inaccurately
- Avoid first-person address when discussing issues that may be perceived as negative (e.g., "A patient in this situation might experience an infection" is preferable to "You may get an infection")
- Some patients, especially females wearing the veil or scarf, may not wish to shake hands with health care personnel of the opposite sex; if gloves are worn, physical contact may be permissible
- Some patients may not make eye contact with health care personnel of the opposite sex
- Haste may be mistaken for rudeness

Summary of Special Issues in Caring for Arab Americans and American Muslims

- Because the needs of the family come before the needs of the individual, full disclosure and patient autonomy may not be possible
- Document a woman's permission to discuss health care matters with her husband
- Family members sometimes prefer to shield the patient from news about terminal illness
- No one Islamic doctrine covers every medical situation; different religious leaders may make different decisions regarding health care issues
- Wide variations exist in the role and social position of women; some Muslim women have professional careers and active social lives, whereas others rarely leave their homes
- Hospital patients may object to tub baths or request frequent changes of water because of cultural attitudes toward using soiled water
- Patients usually prefer to deal with health care personnel of the same sex
- Prayers should not be interrupted; do not walk in front of a patient who is praying
- Some patients may not be time-conscious (e.g., late for appointments)
- Mental illness and depression may be considered culturally and religiously taboo
- Higher rate of smoking
- Reluctance to admit to drug addiction
- Special issues surround fasting during Ramadan
- Discussions of sexually transmitted diseases are offensive to many Muslims, but education and screening remain necessary
- Pelvic exams and Pap smears in unmarried women raise issues concerning virginity and therefore require significant discussion
- Generally acceptable medical treatments include IV, blood transfusion, and blood products; unacceptable medical treatments include medicine or other medical products derived from pork (e.g., pork insulin)
- Donation and receipt of organs for transplant from a living donor are usually acceptable as long as the donor's life is not threatened and the donation is not part of the external body (e.g., an eye); whether organs are to be donated or received after death remains a controversial issue, and decisions should be made on an individual basis

REFERENCES

1. Shabbas A, Al-Qazzaz A, eds. Arab World Notebook. Berkeley, CA: Arab World & Islamic Resources; 1989:49-50.

2. Naff A. Becoming American: The Early Arab Immigrant Experience. Carbondale, IL: Southern Illinois University Press; 1993:2-3.

3. Sengstock MC. Detroit's Iraqi-Chaldeans: a conflicting conception of identity. In: Abraham SY, Abraham N, eds. Arabs in the New World. Detroit: Wayne State University Press; 1983:140-1.

4. Nu'man FH. The Muslim Population in the United States: A Brief Statement. Washington, DC: American Muslim Council; 1992:13.

5. Zogby J. Arab America Today: A Demographic Profile of Arab Americans. Washington, DC: Arab American Institute; 1990.

6. *Ibid.*, pp 19-30.

7. *Ibid.*, p 16.

8. *Ibid.*, p 7.

9. ACCESS Cardiovascular Disease Risk Reduction Project. Dearborn: Michigan Public Health Institute, Resource Center for Cardiovascular Health; 1997-1998.

10. Sachedina A. Living Islam in America [Lecture Series on *Ashura'a*]. Dearborn Heights, MI: Islamic House of Wisdom; 1998.

11. Islam: the essentials [statement prepared by the Islamic Foundation]. In Ahmad K, ed. Islam: Its Meaning and Message, 2nd ed. London: The Islamic Foundation; 1976:21-6.

12. Matar NI. Islam for Beginners. New York: Writers and Readers Publishing; 1992:51-5.

13. Siblani MK. Islam and the Muslim Patient: Impact of Religion and Culture on Health Care Delivery. Dearborn, MI: Oasis Health & Educational Services; 1998:24.

14. Gostin LO. Informed consent, cultural sensitivity, and respect for persons. JAMA. 1995;274:844-5.

15. Sengstock MC. Care of the elderly within Muslim families. In: Aswad BC, Bilge B, eds. Family and Gender among American Muslims: Issues Facing Middle Eastern Immigrants and Their Descendants. Philadelphia: Temple University Press; 1996:271-97.

16. Ethnic Medicine Guide. Harborview Medical Center, University of Washington; 1995. This online reference can be found at http://ethnomed.org/.

17. Nydell MK. Understanding Arabs: A Guide for Westerners. Yarmouth, ME: Intercultural Press; 1987:103-7.

18. *Ibid.*, p 25.

19. Meleis AI. The Arab American in the health care system. Am J Nurs. 1981;81:1180-3.

20. Handwerker WP. Cultural diversity, stress, and depression: working women in the Americas. J Women's Health Gend Based Med. 1999;8:1303-11.

21. Goetzel RZ. The relationship between modifiable health risks and health care expenditures: an analysis of the multi-employer HERO health risk and cost database. The Health Enhancement Research Organization (HERO) Research Committee. J Occup Environ Med. 1998;40:843-54.

22. Pickthall MM, translator. Surah 5, Verse 3. In: The Meaning of the Glorious Koran: An Explanatory Translation. New York: Penguin Books; 1992:

23. Siblani MK. *Op. cit.*, p 27.

24. Zaid BA. Fiqh an-Nawazil. Riyadh: Maktabah ar-Rushd; 1407 AH. 1988;1:215-36.

7

Caring for Immigrants

BARBARA OGUR, MD

Immigration is the cornerstone of this nation's existence. In recent years, globalization of the world's economy, ecological changes, and regional wars have disrupted the economies of many poorer countries, which in turn has contributed to a steady increase in the number of immigrants to the United States. Immigrants come largely from Central and South America, the Caribbean, Asia, and, more recently, from countries of the former Soviet Union (1). In 1999, almost 26 million Americans identified themselves as foreign-born; more than one quarter of these immigrants had come to the United States within the past ten years (2).

The Bureau of the Census provides data on the region of birth of foreign-born United States residents. These data give one a picture of immigration trends over the past century but may undercount certain immigrant groups by as much as 20% to 40% (3). The Immigration and Naturalization Service (INS), using multiple data sets, including overstays by foreign visitors, deaths of resident undocumented immigrants, Census data, and other statistics, estimated that in 1996 approximately 5 million undocumented immigrants were residing in the United States, with this population growing by about 250,000 annually. The INS data provide a picture of undocumented immigrant communities by country of origin and state of residence within the United States (Table 7-1) (4).

Census data do not distinguish between *immigrants,* individuals who emigrate from their home country because of perceived economic advantages, professional advancement, or desire to join other family members, and *refugees,* who "owing to well-founded fear of being persecuted for reasons of race, religion, nationality, or membership in a particular group of political opinion are outside the country of their nationality" (5). This distinction is important, because refugees are more likely than immigrants to experience profound infectious, nutritional, and psychological problems (6,7).

Table 7-1   Estimated Illegal Immigrant Population: Top 20 Countries of Origin and States of Residence (October 1996)

Country of Origin		State of Residence	
Mexico	2,700,000	California	2,000,000
El Salvador	335,000	Texas	700,000
Guatemala	165,000	New York	540,000
Canada	120,000	Florida	350,000
Haiti	105,000	Illinois	290,000
Philippines	95,000	New Jersey	135,000
Honduras	90,000	Arizona	115,000
Nicaragua	70,000	Massachusetts	85,000
Poland	70,000	Virginia	55,000
Bahamas	70,000	Washington	52,000
Colombia	65,000	Colorado	45,000
Ecuador	55,000	Maryland	44,000
Dominican Republic	50,000	Michigan	37,000
Trinidad & Tobago	50,000	Pennsylvania	37,000
Jamaica	50,000	New Mexico	37,000
Pakistan	41,000	Oregon	33,000
India	33,000	Georgia	32,000
Dominica	32,000	District of Columbia	30,000
Peru	30,000	Connecticut	29,000
Korea	30,000	Nevada	24,000
Other	744,000	Other	330,000

From Immigration and Naturalization Service data.

Census data also do not completely capture the situation of people who emigrate due to natural disaster or devastating economic conditions, famine, or war. The largest refugee groups entering the United States over the past 20 years have been from Southeast Asia, Central America, and the former Soviet Union; most of these refugees left their countries because of war or revolution.

Medical care of immigrants often presents special challenges. Differential diagnosis must include diseases endemic to the patient's country of origin and sometimes requires consideration of infectious diseases that may present threats to the public's health. The process of immigration itself may cause illness. People driven to emigrate by violence, economic hardships, or natural disasters have often undergone tremendous stress if not physical injury; they often have unstable or disrupted family and social situations; and they may encounter economic or discriminatory barriers that prevent them from re-establishing a nurturing community in the United States.

Immigrants frequently work in low-paying, dangerous jobs, often without knowledge of or without recourse to occupational safety protections. Cultural variations in the understanding of disease causation and treatment, language differences, and discordant role expectations make communication complex. Access to care may be severely limited by immigration status, limitations on services for even documented immigrants, lack of insurance benefits in entry-level jobs, unavailability of linguistically appropriate services, or overtly discriminatory policies.

Establishing Differential Diagnoses

Recognizing "Exotic" Pathogens

Physicians may be challenged to include differential diagnostic possibilities of which they have only textbook knowledge, without the experience to recognize atypical presentations of diseases endemic in the patient's country of origin. Recent travel history may not suggest all possible infectious pathogens, because parasitic illness may persist in quiescent form for years and infectious sources (e.g., food, contact with others more recently arrived in the United States) may spread disease (Case 7-1).

Familiarity with "exotic" pathogens has become increasingly important even for physicians who see few immigrants. For example, cholera, which initially re-emerged in epidemic proportions in the Western Hemisphere in Peru after nearly a century's absence, has been isolated from oysters in beds along the Gulf Coast (8). Local transmission of malaria has been documented in San Diego (9), Houston, New Jersey, and, in New York, Queens and Suffolk County, likely reflecting both the new introduction of infection from immigrants and endemic spread (10,11). Similarly, the endemic spread

---

**CASE 7-1   A 26-YEAR OLD EL SALVADORIAN MALE WHO EATS
UNHEALTHY IMPORTED CHEESE**

JR is a 26-year-old male from El Salvador who has not traveled outside the United States in three years. He presents to the hospital complaining of headache and fevers up to 103°F for 10 days before admission. He has not had contact with any recent immigrants, but about 2 weeks ago he ate some special El Salvadorian cheese that had been smuggled in for him. Blood cultures were positive for Salmonella typhi.

---

neurocysticercosis (12) has been demonstrated, with likely initial introduction by immigrant domestic workers. Typhoid fever outbreaks in the United States have increased, with at least one outbreak traced to a recent immigrant (13).

Taking the History

Several historical features can assist physicians in differential diagnostic reasoning. Of major importance is the geographic region from which the immigrant comes, including the climate and biological habitat. For example, malaria species with resistance to chloroquine, and even to mefloquine and sulfadoxine-pyrimethamine, exist in certain parts of the world. In some countries malaria occurs chiefly in rural areas with heavy rainfall and is uncommon in urban areas.

The Centers for Disease Control and Prevention (CDC) provides a wide range of information about disease prevalence, prevention, and treatment on its Web site (*www.cdc.gov*). Especially important for the physician treating the immigrant patient are its links to health advice for travelers and to the National Center for Infectious Diseases. The World Health Organization (*www.who.org*) and the Pan-American Health Organization (*www.paho.org*) also have valuable statistical data and disease-specific information. Using these resources or recent textbooks (14), physicians can obtain information about diseases prevalent in the immigrant's region of origin. If patients are taking medicines from abroad, the Massachusetts College of Pharmacy's Drug Information Center (617/732-2759), although not specifically an international pharmaceutical resource, can often provide assistance in identifying the substance.

The socioeconomic history can also contribute to differential reasoning. Information about the patient's lifestyle before immigration, and the causes of and process of immigration, can provide insight into possible exposures to contaminated water, to periods of poor nutrition, or to animal and insect reservoirs of certain illnesses (e.g., lice, mosquitoes, rodents, domestic animals). A number of cues may indicate risk for sexually transmitted infection, including long periods of separation from a spouse or, for women in particular, being in regions of conflict or situations of extreme dependency, where forced sexual acts or refusal on the part of men to use condoms may be an issue.

Length of time in the United States and history of contact with more recent immigrants can be important, because a number of illnesses have short incubation periods and therefore may be considered less likely unless contacts with recent immigrants or products from abroad have occurred.

Common Disease Syndromes of Immigrant Patients

Febrile Illness

Initial evaluation of an acutely ill immigrant patient may require empiric treatment and isolation procedures. Severely ill immigrants at risk for falciparum malaria should be treated pending evaluation. Clearly, physicians should also consider infections that are common in nonimmigrants (e.g., urinary tract infections, community-acquired respiratory infections).

Certain febrile illnesses are public health concerns. Patients presenting with hemorrhagic fever within 3 weeks of immigration should be isolated due to the potential human-to-human transmission of certain viral hemorrhagic fevers (15). Patients with possible pulmonary tuberculosis should be isolated in negative pressure rooms. Body fluid precautions should be used for patients with hepatitis and enteric pathogens. Specific instructions about types of isolation precautions are available on the Internet (*www.cdc.gov/health/diseases*).

Duration of time since potential exposure may be very helpful in orienting differential diagnostic thinking (Table 7-2). Another method for characterizing febrile illnesses that may aid in differential thinking is to organize them by commonly associated signs and symptoms (Table 7-3) (16).

Table 7-2   Typical Incubation Periods for Tropical Infectious Diseases

Short (<10 Days)	Intermediate (10-21 Days)	Prolonged (>21 Days)
• Arbovirus infection (dengue, West Nile, Rift Valley, Lassa, *Phlebotomus*, Oropouche, etc.)	• Typhus	• Amebiasis
	• Typhoid fever	• Viral hepatitis
	• Q fever	• Tuberculosis
	• Some hemorrhagic fevers	• Malaria
• Yellow fever	• Malaria	• Acute schistosomiasis
• Rickettsial infection	• Leptospirosis	• Filariasis
• *Yersinia pestis*	• Borreliosis	• Leishmaniasis
• Nontyphoidal salmonellosis		• Meliodiosis
		• Paragonimiasis
• Toxigenic *E. coli*		• Strongyloidiasis
• *Campylobacter* enteritis		• Actinomyces
		• Rabies
• Leptospirosis		• Trypanosomiasis
		• Brucellosis

Adapted from Strickland GT. Fever in travelers. In: Hunter's Tropical Medicine, 8th ed. Philadelphia: WB Saunders; 2000:1050.

Studies of causes of fever among American travelers returning from the tropics provide some insight. However, because immigrants usually come from different socioeconomic circumstances and have different levels of acquired immunity to endemic diseases, these are not clearly comparable populations. The most common tropical infections in travelers are malaria, enteric fever, viral hepatitis, and dengue (17). Dengue is underdiagnosed and should be considered in patients with fever, arthralgias, headaches, with or without rash, who have a history of travel to the tropics (including Puerto Rico and Mexico) within the preceding 3 weeks (18). In instances of severe febrile illness, physicians should consider early consultation with an infectious disease specialist to ensure that all relevant diagnostic procedures are performed before initiating treatments that may limit the usefulness of cultures.

Malaria

Malaria is the leading parasitic cause of death worldwide, with an estimated 100 million cases per year and several million deaths (19). In 1998, 1611 cases of malaria were reported to the CDC (20), most occurring in immigrants or travelers returning from endemic areas. Previous infection with malaria does not confer protective immunity. It does result in partial

Table 7-3   Common Presentations and Febrile Illnesses of Immigrants

Symptom or Finding	Differential Diagnoses
Hemorrhagic complications	Yellow fever, malaria, dengue, arbovirus infections, arenavirus infections, *Hantavirus,* Junin virus, Ebola and Marburg viruses
Prominent pulmonary symptoms	*Cavitary disease:* tuberculosis, melioidosis, paragonimiasis, histoplasmosis, blastomycosis, coccidioidomycosis
	Infiltrates: pulmonary cycle of parasites (ascariasis, hookworm, strongyloidiasis, toxocariasis, schistosomiasis, *Wuchereria bancrofti, Brugia malayi*), *Yersinia pestis,* leptospirosis
	Cor pulmonale: schistosomiasis
	Localized mass: amebic abscess, *Echinococcus* cysts
	Pleural disease: amebic abscess, tuberculosis
	ARDS: leptospirosis, *Hantavirus*
Jaundice	Hepatitis A, B, D, E; leptospirosis
Prominent skin findings	*Rash:* dengue, measles, meningiococcus, rickettsial infection, typhoid fever, syphilis, viral exanthems, borreliosis, bartonellosis
	Ulcers: anthrax, chagas, leishmaniasis, LGV, African trypanosomiasis, rickettsial infection, yaws, syphilis
	Localized swelling: chagas, pinta, gnathostomiasis, loiasis, myiasis
	Conjunctivitis: leptospirosis
Lymphadenopathy	Brucellosis, *Yersinia pestis,* tuberculosis, leptospirosis, meliodosis, disseminated fungal infections, visceral leishmaniasis, filariasis, African and American trypanosomiasis
CNS obtundation	Malaria, rickettsial infection, African trypanosomiasis, meningiococcus, viral hemorrhagic fevers, rabies, leptospirosis, neurocysticercosis

Adapted from Strickland GT. Fevers in travelers. In: Hunter's Tropical Medicine, 8th ed. Philadelphia: WB Saunders; 2000:1051-2.

immunity, which may attenuate and prolong the course. Most immigrants do not have access to malaria prophylaxis. Even when they do, regimens are not 100% effective, particularly in areas of chloroquine or mefloquine resistance such as Southeast Asia and parts of Africa (21).

Diagnosis of malaria may easily be overlooked. Patients may present with nonspecific symptoms of fever, chills, vomiting, anorexia, and headache, resulting in initial misdiagnosis of gastroenteritis or hepatitis (22). Malaria has been described as the "great mimic", because the classic periodicity may not be present and signs and symptoms for each patient may differ. The incubation period varies from 12 to 14 days for *Plasmodium falciparum* to 35 days for *P. malariae* but may be much longer (months to years) in patients with partial immunity (23). Partially immune individuals may have parasitemia without symptoms (24,25).

Early diagnosis and treatment of falciparum malaria is critical because of its significant mortality. Potential sequelae include cerebral infection, acute renal failure, noncardiogenic pulmonary edema, hypoglycemia, and shock. Women in the second and third trimester of pregnancy and in the early post-partum period are both more susceptible to malaria and more likely to experience severe illness, including maternal mortality, stillbirth, and premature delivery (26).

Diagnosis is usually made through the examination of Giemsa-stained thick and thin smears of peripheral blood, with the first smear positive in 95% of cases. Smears should be examined every 6 to 12 hr over 48 hr due to the cyclical nature of the parasitemia. Newer monoclonal antibody tests appear to have sensitivity equal to the screening of blood smears. Appropriate treatment depends upon the type of malaria and typical antimicrobial resistance patterns in the geographic area of origin (27). In seriously ill patients empiric treatment should be started without awaiting confirmatory tests.

Tuberculosis

Among foreign-born persons residing in the United States the incidence rate for active tuberculosis is almost quadruple the rate for native residents, representing 39% of reported cases in 1997. The CDC has determined that those at highest risk of developing active TB are older immigrants (especially those ≥55 years of age), recent immigrants from countries with high rates of the disease (the Philippines, Vietnam, Haiti, Korea, and sub-Saharan Africa), and immigrants from these high-risk areas who have been in the United States less than 5 years (28).

Although previous guidelines recommended prophylaxis for asymptomatic patients with normal chest x-rays only if they were younger than 35 years old, recent revisions have stressed the need for prophylaxis for any individuals at increased risk, including recent immigrants from countries with a high prevalence of TB (29). This is an important argument for ensuring that all immigrant patients who have been in the United States for less than 5 years receive primary care with PPD testing.

Immigrants and refugees who want to enter the United States must have been screened for TB overseas within 1 year of entry. Applicants already in the United States must be screened and found free of infectious TB before they can adjust their immigration status. Of those screened overseas, 3% to 14% of the approximately 6000 Class B1 (smear negative but x-ray compatible with active disease) immigrants and 0.4% to 4% of the 12,000 Class B2 (x-ray compatible with inactive disease) immigrants who enter the country each year develop active TB after arrival in the United States. These individuals are at high risk for reactivation and are candidates for preventive therapy. Preventive therapy is recommended for persons from high-risk areas with PPD skin-test reactions ≥10 mm even if they have negative chest x-rays and regardless of whether they have received BCG vaccination.

Because it is prevalent worldwide, and because its manifestations are so varied, tuberculosis must be included in the differential diagnosis of any serious or chronic febrile illness. Compared with U.S.-born patients, a higher percentage of foreign-born patients have extrapulmonary TB only. Drug-resistance rates are higher among foreign-born populations because medications may be available without prescription and because many patients cannot afford to pay for a full course of therapy. Levels of INH resistance are higher among TB patients born in Vietnam (18.3%), the Philippines (14.7%), and Mexico (9.8%) than among U.S.-born TB patients (6.4%) (30). The outcome of TB treatment is slightly better for foreign-born patients than for U.S.-born patients. Among the foreign-born, levels of completion vary by country of origin, but, among the major immigrant groups, completion rates equal or exceed those among U.S.-born patients.

In the United States, HIV infection has not played a major role in TB cases among foreign-born persons. In fact, whereas 19% of U.S.-born patients with active TB were HIV+, only 6% of foreign-born patients had HIV co-infection (31). The low overall incidence of HIV among foreign-born persons with TB may be partly attributable to the federal law prohibiting persons with HIV infection from applying for overseas immigration. Recent studies conducted in South Florida, however, indicated higher rates of HIV co-infection in Florida immigrants with active TB, perhaps reflecting the presence of more undocumented immigrants and asylum seekers (who do not go through screening in their home countries before immigrating). For immigrant patients between the ages of 25 and 44 with active TB for whom HIV results were available (59%), 80% of Haitian immigrants, 67% of Cubans, and 43% of other Latin Americans were HIV+ (31).

Diarrhea

Acute Diarrhea

As in acute febrile illness, when evaluating a person with acute diarrhea it is important to assess several key historical features. Important details include the length of time in the United States, contact with recent immigrants or imported foods, and, if recently arrived, possible exposures during the immigration process. Median duration of acute diarrhea is 3 or 4 days, with only 10% of cases lasting longer than 1 week. Approximately 15% of patients experience vomiting, and 2% to 10% may have accompanying fever, bloody stools, or both (32). As in American-acquired or travel-associated acute diarrhea, most cases are self-limited and caused by infections with enterotoxigenic *Escherichia coli, Salmonella, Shigella, Campylobacter jejuni,* and enteric viruses. In most cases, antibiotic treatment is not indicated and may even prolong the carrier state. However, in severe *Shigella* dysentery, amebic dysentery, and *Vibrio cholerae* infection, antibiotic treatment should be given. Patients with voluminous diarrhea or bloody diarrhea should have bacterial cultures, stools for ova and parasites, and *Clostridium difficile* assays if antibiotics have already been tried.

Chronic Diarrhea

Diarrhea persisting more than 4 weeks requires more extensive evaluation. Accompanying symptoms of bloody stools and/or malabsorption may assist in developing the differential diagnosis. Whereas in the United States diarrhea persisting more than 4 weeks is commonly noninfectious, immigrants frequently are exposed to infectious sources. Therefore work-up should include fecal leukocytes, Sudan stain for fat, fecal antigen testing for *Giardia,* three specimens for ova and parasite examination, and special examination for cryptosporidium, isospora, microsporidia and cyclospora (Table 7-4).

Chronic amebiasis may present in the same manner as inflammatory bowel disease, clinically, endoscopically, and radiographically. Because corticosteroids may result in fulminant amebic colitis, immigrant patients with

Table 7-4	Differential Diagnosis of Diarrhea
Chronic Bloody Diarrhea	Diarrhea Associated with Malabsorption
• Parasitic infections (amebiasis, Trichuris) • Campylobacter infection	• Tropical sprue • Giardia • Strongyloides • Cryptosporidium • Isospora • Filariasis with lymphatic obstruction • Chagas' disease with pseudoobstruction or bacterial overgrowth • Tropical enteropathy • HIV enteropathy

presumptive inflammatory bowel disease should have stool cultures and serology to rule out amebiasis before initiating corticosteroid treatment (33).

Chronic giardiasis is common, with prevalence rates of 20% to 30% in the developing world. Because detection of cysts or trophozoites may be difficult, many experts recommend empiric treatment for patients with the typical symptoms of diarrhea (bloating, abdominal discomfort, nausea, flatulence, fatigue), even if stools are negative (34). After effective treatment, symptoms may resolve gradually over several weeks, due to secondary lactose intolerance induced by the infection.

Tropical sprue, a disease manifesting with chronic diarrhea, malabsorption, and deficiencies of folate and vitamin B_{12}, may occur in immigrants from tropical regions, particularly Haiti, Puerto Rico, the Dominican Republic, India, and Southeast Asia. It is rarely seen in Africa. Definitive diagnosis is by small bowel biopsy. Although an infectious etiology has yet to be confirmed, treatment with a prolonged course of tetracycline and folic acid is usually effective.

Hepatitis A Virus Infection

Hepatitis A is highly endemic in the developing world, including Central and South America, the Middle East, Africa, and Asia, and moderately endemic in countries of the former Soviet Union. It is generally acquired in childhood, has a mild clinical course, and results in protective immunity. With increasing development, acquisition of infection may be delayed until adulthood, with the potential for more serious disease.

Hepatitis B Virus Infection

Researchers divide the world into areas of high, intermediate, and low endemicity for hepatitis B virus (HBV). Sub-Saharan Africa, Asia east of the Indian sub-continent, the Pacific Basin, the Amazon Basin, the Arctic Rim, Asian Republics of the former Soviet Union, portions of the Middle East, Asia Minor and the Caribbean have high endemicity, with 50% to 95% of the population becoming infected with the virus during childhood. Eight to fifteen percent of the general population become chronic carriers. In these regions liver cancer caused by hepatitis B is a significant cause of cancer death in men.

In areas of intermediate endemicity, 30% to 50% of the population have evidence of previous infection. Two to five percent of the population become chronic carriers. These areas include parts of southern and eastern Europe, the Middle East, western Asia through the Indian subcontinent and parts of Central and South America (35). In these areas, acute hepatitis with jaundice is more commonly seen, because a substantial portion of infection occurs in older adolescents and adults who generally have more prominent symptoms of acute clinical disease than children with acute infection.

Hepatitis C Virus Infection

Prevalence of hepatitis C infection varies by region, with WHO estimates of 5.3% in Africa, 1.7% in the Americas, 4.6% in the eastern Mediterranean, 1.03% in Europe, 2.15% in Southeast Asia, and 3.9% in the western Pacific (36). In developing nations, inadequate screening of blood products for transfusion and inadequately sterilized equipment are the major sources of transmission, as illustrated by the prevalence rate of 15% to 20% in Egypt, attributable to an aggressive program of potassium antimony tartrate injections against schistosomiasis conducted until the 1980s (37).

Parasitic and Protozoan Infections

A number of studies have indicated that there is no clear relationship between symptoms and parasitic infection. Though screening data show prevalence rates ranging from 11% to 61% in patients immigrating from developing countries and gastrointestinal symptoms are common in immigrant patients, studies have not shown patients with parasites to be significantly more likely to have gastrointestinal symptoms nor are patients with symptoms more likely to have parasites (38,39). Most authorities recommend, however, that immigrants with gastrointestinal symptoms undergo screening for parasitic infection.

Most intestinal parasites do not replicate within humans but require a cycle of passage through soil or other hosts for cysts or larvae to mature. Thus humans must be reinfected from contaminated sources and, without exposure, will ultimately clear their infections. *Strongyloides stercoralis, Giardia, Entamoeba histolytica,* and *Hymenolepsis nana* are exceptions, because they are capable of replication within the human host and thus may persist for years. Other parasites, while not capable of completing their life cycles in humans, can persist for long periods of time and result in complications; *Taenia solium,* for instance, produces eggs that can be transmitted to others and cause complications such as neurocysticercosis.

The reason for treating intestinal parasitic infection is not simply to eradicate symptoms. Serious complications are possible, though rare. *Strongyloides,* particularly in the setting of concomitant depression of host immunity due to malnutrition, malignancy, or the use of immunosuppressives or corticosteroids, can disseminate, causing serious septicemia with a significant mortality. *Ascaris,* besides causing pulmonary eosinophilic syndromes, can migrate into the biliary tree or bowel, resulting in cholecystitis, pancreatitis, intrahepatic abscesses, and acute appendicitis (40).

Examining stool specimens is an important diagnostic test. Generally, three specimens are collected, which is quite sensitive for most parasites except for *Entamoeba histolytica, Strongyloides,* and *Schistosomiasis.* Specimens should be examined when fresh. If delay in transport is unavoidable, samples may be preserved in two portions, one of polyvinyl alcohol, which fixes protozoan trophozoites, and the other of 5% or 10% buffered formaldehyde, which preserves ova and cysts. Serologic tests are available to detect *Strongyloides, Schistosomiasis,* and amebiasis. There is no evidence to support routine use of serologic tests in screening asymptomatic immigrants. Serology for *Schistosomiasis* cannot differentiate between previous and acute infection. Serologic testing for *Strongyloides* may be helpful in the evaluation of unexplained eosinophilia and the detection of asymptomatic infection in patients at risk for immunosuppression and the development of disseminated strongyloidiasis.

Enteric ameba and flagellates (*Entamoeba hartmanni, Entamoeba coli, Entamoeba polecki, Endolimax nana, Iodamoeba butschlii, Entamoeba dispar, Trichomonas hominis, Chilomastix mesnili*) may be detected but are not pathogenic and do not require treatment. There is disagreement as to whether *Blastocystis hominis* is a pathogen. Some authorities recommend treatment if symptoms are present (41). Because the presence of nonpathogenic species indicates contact with contaminated water sources, patients with on-going symptoms should undergo further investigation to identify pathogenic species such as *Cryptosporidia, Isospora, Microsporida,* and *Cylospora.*

Given the availability of reasonably safe and effective treatments, some experts suggest that cost-effectiveness analysis supports the presumptive administration of albendazole to all immigrants at risk for parasitosis (42), although this is not a universal standard of care. Albendazole appears to have efficacy against *Giardia.* Albendazole is contraindicated in pregnant women.

Schistosomiasis

Acute schistosomiasis, an illness characterized by fever, myalgias, lethargy, eosinophilia, and sometimes by cercarial dermatitis, may be seen in immigrants previously naïve to the infection, with an incubation period of 35 to 40 days after contact with contaminated fresh water. Long-term complications of chronic schistosomiasis depend upon the site of deposition of eggs by the adult worms. Intestinal schistosomes (*Schistosoma japonicum, S. mansoni, S. intercalatum, S. mekongi*), found in Africa, South America, the Caribbean, the Middle East, and the Far East inhabit the mesenteric veins. Complications include portal hypertension, caused by the deposition of eggs, with resultant fibrosis in the hepatic venules, and bloody diarrhea and colonic polyps, caused by egg deposition in mesenteric venules. Urinary schistosomiasis is typically caused by *S. haemotobium,* which is found in Africa and the Middle East. Adult worms residing in the veins surrounding the urinary bladder result in obstructive uropathy, hematuria, and possibly bladder cancer. Rarely, schistosomal eggs may lodge in the pulmonary capillary beds, causing pulmonary hypertension, or may enter the central nervous system via the vertebral venous plexus, with complications including transverse myelitis and space-occupying lesions (43).

Negative serologic testing excludes the diagnosis of schistosomiasis. Positive serology indicates previous, but not necessarily active, infection. Stool, urine, or biopsy detection of the organism is usually necessary to make the diagnosis.

Eosinophilia

Parasitic infection is a major cause of eosinophilia worldwide, chiefly associated with helminthic infections. More rarely, infection with *Isospora* or *Dientamoeba fragilis,* TB, coccidioidomycosis or leprosy, or infestation with ectoparasites such as scabies may cause eosinophilia. In general, parasites elicit eosinophilia during migration through host tissues, with more vigorous eosinophilia manifested at initial infection, in non-immune hosts, and during tissue migratory phases of the parasite's life cycle.

When eosinophilia is found, careful geographic history, medication history, and elicitation of accompanying symptoms may help to narrow possible differential diagnostic considerations. Basic work-up should include three stool specimens for ova and parasites, urinalysis with microscopic examination of sediment (hematuria may suggest schistosomiasis), PPD testing, and chest x-ray if there are respiratory symptoms to assess for infiltrates representing the migration of parasites through the lungs.

Negative stools or tissue biopsy specimens do not preclude the presence of parasitic infection, because eosinophilia may precede the development of a latent infection (when "offspring" of the adult parasites can be detected). Eosinophilia may develop or increase following treatment and may last for months after eradication of infection. If eosinophilia persists, and stool examinations are negative, serologic evaluation for strongyloidiasis, toxocariasis, filariasis, and schistosomiasis may be helpful if the geographic history is consistent. Providers should also consider giving a trial of empiric treatment with anti-helminth therapy.

Dyspepsia, Cramping, and Flatulence

Dyspeptic symptoms are common in immigrant patients, with reported rates of 60% to 100% (44). In addition, immigrants have higher rates of *H. pylori* infection. Most people from the developing world are infected during childhood, with most studies of adults in the developing world showing prevalence rates of over 50% (45). However, no association between *H. pylori* infection and dyspeptic symptoms has been found. In the absence of clear evidence that eradication of *H. pylori* is associated with improvement of symptoms or decreased incidence of serious sequelae such as stomach cancer, there is insufficient evidence to warrant *H. pylori* screening of immigrant patients with dyspepsia.

Physicians should consider chronic giardiasis in patients with chronic, nonspecific upper abdominal symptoms. Chronic giardiasis is characterized by loose stools, steatorrhea, weight loss, malabsorption, malaise, fatigue, abdominal cramping, borborygmi, flatulence and burping—all of which may wax and wane over months—, accompanied by an acquired lactose intolerance. Because *Giardia*, like other intestinal parasites, is excreted intermittently, three stool specimens are needed to yield a sensitivity of 90%. Antigen assays can improve the sensitivity.

HIV Infection

Although an estimated 33.4 million people are estimated to be living with HIV/AIDS worldwide, 95% of whom live in developing countries (46), the majority of HIV/AIDS cases in the United States are among the native-born. It is likely that this reflects two major aspects of federal immigration policy: the exclusion of legal immigrants who are HIV infected and the preponderance of undocumented immigration from countries that, as yet, do not have high rates of HIV disease.

HIV-infected immigrants are more likely to develop co-infections with infectious diseases prevalent in their countries of origin, such as TB, chronic diarrheal illness from *Microsporidia* and *Isospora,* and cryptococcosis. Kaposi's sarcoma, pneumocystis pneumonia, *Mycobacterium avium* complex, and lymphomas are relatively less common in immigrants than in patients from the United States.

Caring for HIV-infected immigrant patients presents significant challenges. Once HIV is diagnosed, patients usually are not able to obtain full legal permanent residency or citizenship, and thus frequently do not qualify for full Medicaid benefits. While individual state programs may fill some of this gap by providing medicines and some services without requiring evidence of immigration status, comprehensive services are not uniformly available.

Stigmatization of those with HIV infection may be very severe in immigrant communities. Patients from other countries may mistrust the diagnosis, believing that health providers in the United States stereotypically consider certain ethnic groups at increased risk for HIV. For many immigrants, the association of HIV infection with homosexuality, sexual promiscuity, and injection-drug use, combined with beliefs about possible contagion through ordinary contact, may jeopardize their fragile social support networks. Immigrant patients may try to avoid disclosure of HIV+ status to providers and to family members, and they may be reluctant to use interpreters or community advocates, fearing that their diagnosis will be disclosed to a tight-knit local immigrant community. Providers working with patients in whom HIV is a diagnostic possibility must use care in communicating this concern. Seeking assistance in pre-test counseling from a skilled HIV educator knowledgeable about the patient's culture can be very useful. Local health departments can provide assistance in locating such individuals. Family members or friends should never be used as interpreters for discussing HIV-related issues, unless the patient has given clear consent.

Cancer

Breast cancer incidence rates are highest in North America and northern Europe (70 to 90 per 100,000), intermediate in eastern and southern Europe and South America (40 to 60 per 100,000), and lowest in central and tropical South America, Africa, and Asia (<40 per 100,000). Similarly, colorectal cancers are more prevalent in the United States, with lower rates in northern and western Europe, and even lower in Africa, Asia, and Latin America (47). Immigrant populations tend to have breast, colorectal, and prostate cancer rates that are higher than those in their countries of nativity and lower than those in their host countries (48). The higher risk of cancer after immigration may be due to exposure to different risk factors or adoption of high-risk behaviors after immigrating.

Stomach cancer rates have been declining by 2% to 4% annually in most of the world; this has been attributed to improved methods of food preservation. Rates remain higher in immigrants, however, with the highest rates in immigrants from Japan, followed by Eastern Europe, and parts of Latin America. Although the association between acquisition of *H. pylori* infection at an early age and the development of stomach cancer appears clear, and several authors' models suggest the possibility of benefit from treatment (49), there is no clear evidence that eradication of infection decreases the risk of stomach cancer.

Lung cancer rates in immigrants, as in United States natives, are directly associated with exposure to tobacco and occupational hazards.

Primary liver cancer is directly associated with chronic infection with hepatitis B and C viruses. The geographic areas at highest risk are eastern

Asia, with age-adjusted incidence rates from 27.6 to 36.6 per 100,000 men, Middle Africa (20.8 to 38.1 per 100,000 men), and some countries in western Africa (30 to 48 per 100,000 men), as compared to rates below 5 per 100,000 men in northern Europe and the Caucasian populations of North and South America. Rates among men are 1.5 to 3 times those among women. The combined effects of persistent HBV or HCV infections account for over 80% of primary liver cancer worldwide (50) and represent an important area for potential prevention.

Screening for Disease and Health Maintenance Interventions

A number of programs have screened immigrants for disease. Results from some recent reports are summarized in Table 7-5. Several works provide a detailed breakdown of disease prevalence in immigrants from specific areas of the world (68-70). Immigrants who have been screened abroad must be certified as

1. Having no communicable diseases of public health significance, including HIV, active tuberculosis, infectious syphilis, chancroid, gonorrhea, granuloma inguinale, lymphogranuloma venereum, and leprosy
2. Having documentation of vaccination against vaccine-preventable diseases as recommended by the Advisory Committee for Immunization Practices
3. Free of physical or mental disorders or associated behavior harmful to him/herself or others
4. Free of drug abuse or addiction

Specific Screening Internventions

In addition to age- and gender-specific recommendations, immigrant patients should have several specific screening interventions.

Purified Protein Derivative

All immigrants from countries with high prevalence of tuberculin positivity should have PPD screening. Those with tuberculin reactions >10 mm

Table 7-5   Prevalence of Selected Diseases in Immigrants Related to Area of Origin

	Southeast Asia (51-55)	Africa (56-59)	Mexico, Central America, South America (60-62)	Haiti (63-66)	Eastern Europe and Former Soviet Union (67)
TB: PPD+	42%-98% (active disease: Tibetans 8%; Vietnamese 2%)	47%-57%	35%-58%	59%-76%; 1.5% active TB	40%-51%; active disease in 0.4% of Russians
Intestinal parasites	11%-100% (lower rates among Vietnamese)	38%-71%	39%-60%; prevalence of parasites among non-farm worker immigrants decreases with years in U.S.	22%-70%	2%-3%; lower in Jewish Russian refugees
HBsAg+	8%-14%	7%-15%	2%->8% in Brazil and Amazon basin		2%-8%
VDRL+	12% (19% among Cambodians)	7%			2% in Russia
Vaccines		100% of Somalians incomplete		5%	19% of 0-19 year-olds lack MMR antibodies; 91% of Bosnians incomplete
Other	• 58% of Montagnard refugees; only 17% with +malaria smears reported fever • Of 400 Southeast Asian refugees, 10%-15% with scabies, 90% moderate-to-severe dental problems, 1% rheumatic heart disease, 2.5% goiters, 10% serious psychiatric problems • 1.4/1000 Vietnamese had leprosy	Ethiopians: 0.8%-2% active malaria; Somalians: 15% active malaria	5% of Nicaraguan and Salvadoran immigrants infected with T. cruzi	7% HIV+; 1.7% +malaria smears with no symptoms	40% higher mortality rate, increased cardiovascular disease in women, and increased cerebrovascular disease in both sexes; diphtheria now epidemic in Russia; 80% of Russian immigrants come from areas most affected by Chernobyl disaster

should have chest radiography and should be offered preventive therapy. Before initiating long-term steroid treatment or other immunosuppressive therapies, physicians should strongly consider administering anti-tuberculous prophylaxis to immigrants with positive PPDs.

Stools for Ova and Parasites

Immigrants coming from developing countries and from rural areas of the former Soviet Union should have three stools to screen for ova and parasites to prevent the potential serious sequelae of strongyloidiasis and ascariasis.

Hepatitis A Antibody

Immigrants from countries with high rates of hepatitis A and who are likely to return to visit are vulnerable if they are not immune. It is therefore prudent to test for immunity and vaccinate as appropriate.

Hepatitis B Surface Antigen and Antibody

According to the Preventive Services Task Force, screening for hepatitis B infection is cost-effective in groups with an HBV marker prevalence of >20% (71). Immigrants from areas of high and intermediate endemicity should therefore be screened to detect chronic carriers and nonimmune persons so that prophylactic vaccination can be offered. Areas of high endemicity include sub-Saharan Africa, Asia east of the Indian subcontinent, the Pacific basin, the Amazon basin, the Arctic rim, Asian republics of the former Soviet Union, and parts of the Middle East, Asia Minor, and the Caribbean. Areas of intermediate endemicity include parts of southern and eastern Europe, the Middle East, western Asia through the Indian subcontinent, and parts of Central and South America (72). Of critical importance is the screening of women of childbearing age, because perinatal transmission is extremely efficient. From 70% to 90% of mothers positive for both HbsAg and HbeAg will transmit the infection to their infants, with almost all infants becoming chronic carriers (73).

Hepatitis C

Low prevalence rates and low rates of transmission by sexual contact and perinatally do not appear to warrant widespread screening of asymptomatic immigrants for hepatitis C infection. However, patients found to have HCV should be evaluated for the administration of hepatitis A and B vaccines and for possible treatment of active disease.

VDRL Test

All immigrant patients should be screened with a VDRL serologic test.

Immunizations

Most people who immigrate to the United States come without documentation of vaccinations. Even in the best of circumstances, personal vaccination histories are unreliable. Some authorities recommend a full schedule of immunizations for all adult immigrants (74). Vaccination rates and disease prevalence in the patient's country of origin, available through the World Health Organization (*www.who.int/vaccines-documents/DocsPDF00/www542.pdf*), may be helpful in assessing the likelihood that the patient has received adequate vaccination but will not fulfill documentation requirements for school admission or employment.

Polio

Administration of inactivated (parenteral) polio vaccine should be considered in persons who intend to return to regions where the disease is still endemic (Africa, Southeast Asia, and the eastern Mediterranean). Haiti, the Dominican Republic, and Cape Verde experienced outbreaks of polio in 2000 resulting in CDC recommendations for booster doses of vaccine for visitors to those areas (75).

Measles

The risk of acquiring measles in the United States is low; however, measles can be serious in the adult. For this reason, and because very high levels of immunity (93% to 97% of the population) are needed for complete protection from future measles epidemics, it is prudent to administer at least one dose of measles vaccine, preferably two. Routine vaccination in many developing countries, consisting of a single dose at age 9 months, only provides an 85% seroconversion rate (76). The risks of immunizing an already-immune individual are low (77). (No life-threatening adverse effects have been reported in the medical literature.)

Rubella

Congenital rubella is still a major problem in developing countries, two-thirds of which did not routinely vaccinate against rubella before 1997; the prevalence of the disease is not high enough to reliably provide natural immunity. Fourteen outbreaks were reported in the United States in 1996-98, half of them associated with workplaces employing mainly foreign-born workers of Hispanic origin (78). Vaccination with at least one dose of MMR in women of childbearing age is an important preventive strategy.

Tetanus

Almost all cases of tetanus occur in people who have never completed their primary immunization series. Young men and the elderly are the most likely to lack protective antibodies, because they are unlikely to have been included in vaccination campaigns, which focus on the prevention of neonatal tetanus. The Advisory Committee on Immunization Practices of the CDC recommends additional boosters every 10 years, but the American College of Physicians/American Society of Internal Medicine suggests only one at age 50 if primary vaccination can be verified. Very frequent reimmunizations (e.g., three doses in a year) can cause Arthus-type reactions, and 13 cases of peripheral neuropathy have been reported.

Hepatitis B Vaccine

Two large trials are under way in Gambia and China to evaluate the effectiveness of hepatitis B vaccination in the prevention of HBV infection, chronic liver disease, and liver cancer. These two cohorts are being followed over a 30 to 40 year period to assess the effectiveness of HBV vaccination in preventing chronic liver disease and liver cancer. Although WHO has recommended global mass immunization since the early 1980s and about 80 countries have introduced HBV vaccine into their national immunization programs, only an estimated one third of infants at risk are currently being vaccinated, largely due to the cost of the vaccine (79).

The Preventive Services Task Force recommends vaccinating all young adults and anyone at high risk for infection, which would include immigrants likely to return to visit or live in endemically infected areas (Africa, east Asia including the Asian republics of the former Soviet Union, the Pacific and Amazon basins, the Arctic rim, portions of the Middle East,

Asia Minor, and the Caribbean). The elderly, obese, and immunocompromised should have titres after immunization to verify immunity.

Hepatitis A Vaccine

All nonimmune immigrants who anticipate travel to countries with high or intermediate endemicity should be vaccinated against hepatitis A. Particularly at-risk are those who are chronic carriers of HCV, for whom acute hepatitis A infection may cause fulminant hepatitis (80). Testing for hepatitis A antibody before immunizing immigrants from areas with high prevalence reduces vaccination costs (81).

The vaccine has an excellent safety profile.

Varicella Vaccine

Two doses of varicella vaccine are recommended for adults without a clear history of chicken pox. The vaccine can cause rash and fever, so it may be prudent to perform serologic testing. In those who are unlikely to return for follow up visits, however, blind vaccination may be more appropriate.

Conditions Related to Socioeconomic Circumstances of Country of Origin or Refugee Status

When immigration is driven by economic necessity or war, illnesses which are associated with poverty, or which are consequences of trauma or sequelae of minimal or absent public health and primary care interventions, are common. Many immigrants have not had complete immunizations and have had little or no access to screening and preventive health interventions (Case 7-2).

Family disruption during immigration is common. One spouse may make the initial move to find work and housing for the rest of the family. Prolonged separation caused by economic necessity, immigration constraints, or the needs of family members remaining in the country of origin may create social circumstances for nonmonogamous sexual activity, putting partners at risk for sexually transmitted infection and psychological distress.

Rates of domestic violence vary widely between immigrant groups and may be influenced by the process of immigration. Acculturation may attenuate the problem of abuse for immigrants from cultures where wife abuse is

CASE 7-2 A 21-YEAR-OLD DOMINICAN FEMALE WHO ARRIVES IN THE UNITED STATES WITHOUT MEDICAL SCREENING

RC is a 21-year-old immigrant from the Dominican Republic. She arrived in the United States 3 months ago to rejoin her husband, who had come to America to seek employment several years before. He has returned to the Dominican Republic several times for conjugal visits, however. She comes to the physician's office for a check-up after routine testing of her husband discloses a positive serologic test for syphilis. She has not been to a physician in 5 years. She describes severe shortness of breath and intermittent sensations of a rapid, irregular heartbeat. The diagnosis is severe rheumatic mitral stenosis.

common and considered normative; it also intensifies the stresses on immigrant families, which, in some groups, results in increased domestic abuse (82). As a protection for undocumented women, under the Violence Against Women Act of 1994, abused spouses and children of American citizens and legal permanent residents can self-petition for adjustment of status or cancellation of removal and therefore do not have to depend upon an abusing spouse for legalization of their status.

Recent immigration status is not always a predictor of negative outcome. Dietary fat intake and alcohol consumption increase with acculturation (83). Recently arrived Mexican women have fewer low-birth-weight infants than their more acculturated counterparts.

Symptoms associated with histories of violence or deprivation may be less obvious to physicians not aware of conditions in the patient's country of origin. Patients may present with somatic symptoms (Case 7-3); they may be unaware of the connection between traumatic experiences and physical symptoms, reluctant to discuss their traumas for fear of political or social repercussions (84), or directly fearful of governmental representatives or physicians based on past experiences of torture. The medical history, including coming from a region of civil war or totalitarian government, history of residence in prison or refugee camp, loss of multiple family members due to trauma or violence, or symptoms suggestive of post-traumatic stress disorder, may present cues that the patient is a victim of torture (85). Physicians may be called upon to attend to the medical and psychological sequelae of

---

CASE 7-3   A 61-YEAR-OLD EL SALVADORIAN WOMAN WHO HAS SOMATIC COMPLAINTS

MP is a 61-year-old woman who immigrates to the United States in 1988 with her husband and teenage son to protect the latter from enforced enlistment into the El Salvadorian military during the civil war. She is a frequent visitor to her internist, undergoing a series of work-ups for chronic somatic complaints including chest, back, and abdominal pain. Eventually she is diagnosed with somatization disorder. Anti-depressant therapy, individual counseling, and participation in a group for chronically depressed immigrant women only partially improve her condition. In 1996, after the death of her husband, she returns to her town of origin in El Salvador, where a number of family members still live. On a recent visit to America to see her son, she tells her internist that she is off all medications and has few remaining symptoms.

---

violence and to provide information in asylum advocacy cases or human rights testimony (86). In some instances the extent of suffering so far exceeds the treating physician's own life experiences that it may challenge his or her capacity to bear witness (Case 7-4) (87).

Diseases Related to Occupational and Environmental Hazards

United States immigration policy grants a limited number of employment-based visas to people with extraordinary skills. However, most documented immigrants obtain visas based on close family relationships to American citizens or legal permanent residents. Many arrive in the United States without employment skills or, even with skills, without sufficient mastery of English to work in skilled jobs. Thus most immigrants work in unskilled, low-wage, often nonunionized jobs, subject to exposures to toxic and biologic hazards, accidents, and injuries (Case 7-5). Hence taking an occupational history of immigrant patients is recommended (Box 7-1). Immigrant workers report that safety instruction, warning signals on equipment, and educational materials, when available, are in English only.

CASE 7-4 A 23-YEAR-OLD GUATEMALAN WOMAN WHO DENIES SEXUAL ACTIVITY

LR is a 23-year-old Guatemalan woman who presents shortly after immigrating, complaining of headaches, low back pain, inability to sleep, fatigue, and frequent urination. On further questioning it is found that she had spent the preceding 2 months traveling through Mexico and across the Texas border. She has not had her menses since leaving Guatemala but denies sexual activity. When the patient is informed of a positive pregnancy test she discloses that she had been forced to have sexual intercourse as "payment" for being assisted across the border.

DISCUSSION

This patient will benefit from counseling with someone experienced with sexual assault and immigration issues. She should also undergo counseling and testing about sexually transmitted infections including HIV. Lastly, she should be offered counseling regarding pregnancy disposition that respects her culture, religion, and social circumstances.

When immigrant workers sustain occupationally related illness, they lack familiarity with societal resources like workers' compensation and disability or may be reluctant to seek such services for fear of jeopardizing their chance of becoming American citizens or sponsoring family member visa applications. Undocumented workers are even more marginalized, because the Immigration Reform and Control Act of 1986 provides sanctions against employers who hire undocumented employees.

Certain immigrant groups encounter unusually severe occupational and environmental hazards. Immigrant farm workers incur exposures to pesticides, unsanitary living conditions, and poor access to health care, resulting in high rates of parasitic disease and tuberculosis. An expansion of industrial growth along the United States-Mexican border has generated an influx of industrial workers into unincorporated *colonias,* often lacking basic sanitation and straining local public health and health care delivery systems. Lax enforcement or absence of environmental protection laws has resulted in disproportionate pollution of immigrant communities. Ignorant

---

CASE 7-5   A 34-YEAR-OLD ROMANIAN HOUSE PAINTER WHO PRESENTS WITH NAUSEA AND DIZZINESS

SB is a 34-year-old man from Romania who presents with nausea, headaches, and dizziness. Because he is a house painter, a lead level was obtained and found to be elevated. A painting company that recruits temporary workers and is known to recent immigrants as a place to obtain work had recently hired the patient. The company specializes in low-cost exterior painting in an inner-city neighborhood with old housing stock. SB states that it is usual for the temporary workers, mostly non-English speakers, to be given the job of scraping and preparing the building, after which the permanent workers, mostly English-speakers, do the painting. No special equipment is used to protect the workers.

DISCUSSION

It is important to obtain a good occupational history from immigrant patients and to educate them about the hazards of their employment and how they can protect themselves.

---

or fearful of governmental worker protection agencies, undocumented workers from China and other countries work in unhealthy, illegal garment industry sweat-shops in a number of major American cities.

Obstacles to Accessing Health Care

One of the major barriers immigrants face in accessing health care is language. Hospitals and health centers that provide care for immigrants often do not have sufficient resources to provide interpretation in all possible languages, which can result in serious miscommunication (88). Health-care providers should insist upon the availability of trained interpreters and remain sensitive to the dangers of relying on family members or their own limited knowledge of the language (see Chapter 1) (89).

Economic and legislative barriers to accessing care may cause tragic loss and suffering for immigrant patients. Foreign-born patients are twice as

Box 7-1   Occupational History of Immigrant Patients

1. What is the main work you have done over the last 10 years?

2. Where do you work now?

    1st job:

    2nd job:

3. Describe what you do there.

4. Are you exposed to chemicals (including lead and asbestos), dust or fumes, excessive noise, heat, or cold?

    If yes:
    Have you received safety training and information in your own language?

    Do you use any kind of protective equipment?

    Is there adequate ventilation?

5. Do you perform heavy lifting or repetitive movements of your hands or arms? Do you work with dangerous equipment?

    If yes:
    Do you know how to protect yourself from injury?

6. *If problems identified:*

    Are you aware that there are worker protection laws in the United States that protect all workers, even undocumented ones?

Discussion
Physicians can refer patients to specialists in occupational/environmental medicine for assessment, treatment, and assistance in workplace evaluation.

Courtesy of Dr Rose Goldman; revised by the author.

likely to be uninsured as American-born patients (90), with Hispanics under 65 years old (26% uninsured) and particularly Mexican Americans (42% uninsured) having the highest rates. Uninsured patients are less likely to report having a personal physician and less likely to visit their physician regularly than insured patients (91). Undocumented immigrants have an even higher uninsured rate than documented immigrants of the same ethnic group, resulting in high rates of emergency department use. Moreover, data from Florida, where documentation status was collected at the time of admission, suggest that undocumented, uninsured patients, while having a more severe case mix index, have shorter lengths of stay than uninsured residents and citizens (92). Undocumented immigrants may be unaware that they are eligible for programs like public health services and prenatal care and may be fearful of being questioned about income, employment status, or family structure, even in areas where local governments have taken explicit positions to prevent the release of any information to the INS (Cases 7-6 and 7-7) (93).

Documentation status has major implications for an immigrant's ability to access publicly funded health-related services. To add to the complexity, major changes in eligibility occurred with the Personal Responsibility and Work Opportunity Reconciliation Act of 1996 and the Illegal Immigration Reform and Immigrant Responsibility Act of 1996. These laws terminated eligibility for federally funded services for people in a number of categories of immigration status who previously were fully eligible. In addition, they attempted to make federal and state health benefit programs inaccessible to all noncitizens. Fortunately, at present, benefits to documented immigrants have been restored (94). Interested readers are referred to a questionnaire for assessing eligibility (95). Since eligibility criteria are currently in flux, providers should refer patients to local community legal services or to the INS to ensure accuracy; patients with computer access may find information at *www.imminfo.com* (Table 7-6).

Another barrier to care has been the concept of "public charge". Immigrants seeking any type of adjustment of their immigration status or seeking permission for family members to immigrate may be asked to demonstrate that they are not at risk for becoming a public charge. In many cases, immigrants have been asked to present either proof of health insurance or evidence that they have paid for health services out of pocket. In other instances, immigration officials have called hospitals seeking evidence that immigrant patients have received free services, as grounds to deny

CASE 7-6   A 26-YEAR-OLD EL SALVADORIAN WOMAN WHO PRESENTS WITH PYELONEPHRITIS

AT is a 26-year-old woman from El Salvador who presents with pyelonephritis and a right renal calculus. She is referred for shock-wave lithotripsy. Of the three institutions providing this treatment in her metropolitan area, two require payment before treatment is administered while the third only provides treatment for patients receiving primary care within that system. The patient, who speaks no English, is reluctant to change providers, so she does not have the procedure.

One month later AT presents with a second episode of pyelonephritis. This time the consulting urologist offers to remove the stone operatively. She refuses, concerned that the weeks of recuperation required by open incision would result in loss of her minimum-wage job, the only support for her four children living with their grandmother in El Salvador.

Two weeks later AT presents with a third episode of pyelonephritis. Severe gram-negative sepsis requires emergency treatment and hospitilization.

DISCUSSION

Ensuring appropriate care for immigrant patients may require a complicated process of negotiation. First, the provider needs to assess the specific barriers to access:

1. Does the patient understand and accept the treatment being recommended? If not, the assistance of a professional interpreter, community advocate, or family member may be helpful.

2. Does the patient qualify for state or federal medical assistance programs? A social worker can help assess the situation. Undocumented immigrants, who often work at jobs without health insurance, do not qualify for most governmental programs.

3. Are there special services for the indigent and uninsured in the patient's area? If so, how can the patient's access be facilitated? Community-based agencies or social workers often are aware of these resources and may even provide interpreters to accompany patients who do not speak English.

CASE 7-7   A 75-YEAR-OLD SERIOUSLY ILL BARBADIAN WOMAN UNABLE TO AFFORD LASER TREATMENT

EI is a 75-year-old woman from Barbados with long-standing diabetes, hypertension, and peripheral vascular disease. She came to live with her daughter in the United States 5 years earlier, at the time of her left below-knee amputation, unable to manage alone. Two years ago, she developed deteriorating vision secondary to proliferative diabetic retinopathy. Laser treatment was recommended, but the family was unable to afford the pre-payment. The patient was not eligible for Medicaid because she was undocumented. As her vision has failed, she has become increasingly unable to perform the activities of daily living. Her daughter recently quit her full-time job to take care of her mother.

DISCUSSION

Community resources may be available to help in a situation such as this. Some organizations that provide home care services have free care for uninsured individuals. Churches and culturally based organizations may also provide services at no or little cost.

---

applications for adjustment of status. Fear of losing the possibility of adjusting their status or of bringing family to the United States has therefore prevented immigrants from availing themselves of free health care services. In 1999, the federal government clarified its position, declaring that the receipt of health care services would not be deemed evidence for becoming a public charge (96).

Denying immigrant patients access to primary care is not only harmful for immigrant persons. Effective public health relies on integrating primary health care with systems for case-finding and preventive care. Economic barriers to accessing primary care interrupt screening for illness and the delivery of preventive interventions (e.g., for hepatitis B and tuberculosis). Fear of being reported to immigration authorities prevents some undocumented persons from seeking care, thus exposing domestic and work-place contacts (97), and creating the risk of deterioration of chronic medical conditions (98).

Table 7-6	Entitlements Available to Immigrants			
	Individuals Entitled to Full Medicaid Benefits		Individuals Entitled to Emergency or Labor and Delivery Services Only	
United States Citizens	Documented	Undocumented	Documented	Undocumented
• All	• Legal permanent residents ("green card" holders) • Those granted asylum • Refugees • Parolees admitted for 1 year or more • Those granted "withholding of deportation status" • Conditional entrants pursuant to law before 1 April 1980 • Certain battered spouses and children	• None	• Recipients of status under family unit	• Individuals who entered the U.S. illegally • Individuals who entered legally but violated their immigration status

Cross-Cultural Aspects of Care

According to lay theories of illness, ill health may have its cause in the material world, in the social world, in the supernatural world, or in the individual patient himself or herself (99). Immigrant patients may ascribe illness causality to imbalances in the environment (100), to slips in one's own discipline, or to the vengeance of others (101). The perception of illness causality as a metaphysical phenomenon is not limited to immigrant cultures, as moral attributions in diseases like cancer and AIDS are common (102), but specific belief systems differ between cultures. Differences exist in beliefs such as that sugar substitutes, bruises from being hit, microwave ovens, eating pork, eating spicy foods, breast feeding, and antibiotics cause cancer and that getting cancer is like getting a death sentence (103,104).

These lay understandings may determine not only beliefs regarding causality but also appropriate strategies for treatment.

Physicians coming from mainstream American culture may be unaware of the beliefs and practices of their immigrant patients. In particular, cultural beliefs about certain sensitive areas like the role of the family in the care of patients with serious illness (105), the appropriateness of disclosure of serious diagnoses to the patient (106,107), or even the appropriateness of asking questions about personal or intimate subjects may differ significantly (Case 7-8).

In some cultures, relating psychological distress to physical symptoms may be uncommon, leading patients to present more commonly with concerns about the physical symptomatology, that is, with "somatoform" disorders. In addition, immigrant patients may use traditional healing practices or consult traditional healers, relying on herbal medicines, on the use of physical techniques such as cupping or coining, or on ceremonial or spiritual practices. These healing practices may sometimes work as a complement to Western medicine, but at other times may present obstacles to full engagement in treatment.

Significant differences exist between immigrant groups in utilization of Western medicine and/or traditional medicine after immigration. These differences may reflect varying exposures to Western medicine in the country of origin. Increased use of Western medicine also correlates with English proficiency, educational level, and age. It is not clear to what extent beliefs in traditional models of healing are obstacles to accessing Western medical care. Among immigrants, the strongest predictors of lack of preventive service utilization are standard predictors of lack of access: lack of health insurance and lack of a regular doctor. Traditional health beliefs and utilization of traditional health services do not predict lack of services. Immigrant patients, however, report higher levels of satisfaction with care when providers speak their language and come from the same cultural background.

Western physicians, trained in a model that emphasizes professional expertise, may misinterpret culturally influenced illness behavior. Facility in cross-cultural communication is thus not only a skill for developing rapport but also in ensuring accuracy. Physicians unfamiliar with the cultural mores and beliefs of their patient should consult community advocates or interpreters. Other sources of information include state departments of public health. For example, the Massachusetts Department of Public Health, through

---

**CASE 7-8 A 68-YEAR-OLD TERMINALLY ILL HAITIAN WHOSE
DAUGHTER REQUESTS HE NOT BE INFORMED OF
THE GRAVITY OF HIS CONDITION**

---

*JF, a 68-year-old male who is a recent immigrant from Haiti,
presents with a 1-month history of recurrent vomiting, jaundice, and 20-lb weight loss. Diagnostic work-up reveals a mass
in the head of the pancreas, highly suspicious for pancreatic malignancy, with evidence of likely metastatic infiltration of the
liver. The patient speaks no English.*

*During his hospital stay, his adult daughter remains at his bedside to interpret and provide assistance. When the results of the
abdominal CT scan are presented, his daughter implores the
doctors not to disclose the likely diagnosis to her father. She insists that it is not appropriate in Haitian culture for elders to be
told about terminal illness, because it is believed that they
would become despondent and die more quickly. Families considered it their obligation to assume the burden of the knowledge and to take over decision-making.*

DISCUSSION

Although American physicians may find it unethical not to
inform patients of a terminal diagnosis, it is important to
understand the patient's cultural perspective. Insisting upon
informing a patient may be disruptive to cultural norms and
supportive family dynamics and must be handled sensitively.
In this particular instance, when asked how much he
wanted to know about his illness, the patient answered that
he wanted to know if he was going to die, because if he was,
he preferred to return to Haiti. When the daughter heard
this, she was much more comfortable with his being informed of the diagnosis.

---

its Office of Refugee and Immigrant Health, provides brief synopses of the
history, political environment, religions, beliefs about health, and common
health conditions of all major immigrant groups in Massachusetts; Internet
access is available at *www.state.ma.us/dph/orih/orih.htm.*

Summary of High-Risk Conditions and Risk Factors for Disease in Immigrants

Be on the alert for presenting signs of the following conditions. Keep in mind that the history-taking must take into account cultural differences that may otherwise mislead the physician (e.g., reluctance to talk about sexual activity).

High-Risk Conditions

➤ Cancer
- Stomach cancer
- Liver cancer
  Highest risk in immigrants, particularly men, from eastern Asia and mid- and West Africa

➤ Dengue

➤ Diarrhea
- Infections causing acute diarrhea
- Chronic diarrhea
  - ◆ Consider infectious sources rather than the noninfectious sources common in nonimmigrants
  - ◆ Chronic giardiasis is common (prevalence rates of 20%-30% in developing countries)
  - ◆ Tropical sprue is seen in tropical countries, except in Africa

➤ Dyspepsia
- Prevalence rates of 60%-100%
- Consider chronic giardiasis in addition to more common causes

➤ Enteric fever

➤ Environmental hazards (e.g., possible serious pollution in immigrant communities)

➤ Exposure to occupational hazards
- Immigrants who work in unskilled, nonunionized jobs
- Immigrant farm workers

➤ Hemorrhagic fever

➤ Malaria

➤ Measles

➤ Parasitic infections
- Prevalence rates of 11%-61% in developing countries

➤ Polio

(Cont'd.)

➤ Post-traumatic stress disorder (PTSD) (e.g., victims of war or torture)
➤ Pulmonary tuberculosis
  • Highest rates occur in the Philippines, Vietnam, Haiti, Korea, and sub-Saharan Africa, but prevalence is worldwide
  • PPD+ patients should receive preventive therapy against reactivation if from high-prevalence area
  • Drug resistance rates are higher among immigrants
➤ Rubella
➤ Sexually transmitted diseases
  • Separation from spouse remaining in native country among risk factors that increase likelihood of acquiring an STD
  • HIV less common among immigrants
➤ Tetanus
➤ Viral hepatitis
  • Hepatitis A
    ♦ *High endemicity:* Central and South America, Middle East, Africa, Asia
    ♦ *Moderate endemicity:* Former Soviet Union
  • Hepatitis B
    ♦ *High endemicity:* Asia east of the Indian subcontinent, the Pacific basin, the Amazon basin, the Arctic rim, Asian republics of the former Soviet Union, Middle East, Asia Minor, the Caribbean)
  • Hepatitis C

Risk Factors for Disease and Issues to Explore When Taking History

➤ Diseases endemic to the patient's country of origin
➤ Emigration from countries with war, famine, or natural disaster
  • Possible exposure to violence, torture, or rape
  • Increased likelihood of PTSD or family disruption
➤ If recent immigrant, possible exposures en route
➤ Socioeconomic status provides clues to
  • Possible exposure to contaminated water
  • Poor nutrition
  • Exposure to vectors of disease
➤ Risk factors for sexually transmitted diseases
➤ Contact with more recent immigrants who may be carriers of disease
➤ Use of products (e.g., contaminated food) mailed or imported from the patient's native country

Conclusion

In caring for immigrant patients physicians should be aware of the prevalence of diseases in the country of origin (including diseases caused by the social disruption that occurs with immigration), of public policy issues that create barriers to appropriate care, and of the potential for cross-cultural misunderstanding between provider and patient. Mastering the multi-faceted complexity of health care for immigrants requires maintaining a broad diagnostic scope, attending to cultural and psychological aspects of care, and using multi-disciplinary expertise, including interpreters, community advocates, infectious disease specialists, and providers with specific knowledge of the patient's culture.

REFERENCES

1. Immigration and Naturalization Service. Legal Immigration: Fiscal Year 1998. Annual Report 2, July 1999:1-11.
2. Bureau of the Census. Statistical Abstract of the United States: 2000; p 9.
3. Loue S. Defining the immigrant. In: Loue S, ed. Handbook of Immigrant Health. New York: Plenum Press; 1998:19-36.
4. Immigration and Naturalization Service. Illegal Alien Resident Population. www.ins.gov/graphics/aboutins/statistics/illegalalien/index.htm; 12/20/2000.
5. Castillo R., Waitzkin H, Ramirez Y, Escoba JI. Somatization in primary care, with a focus on immigrants and refugees. Arch Fam Med. 1995;4:637-46.
6. Toole MJ, Waldman RJ. Refugees and displaced persons. JAMA. 1993;270:600-5.
7. Ackerman LK. Health problems of refugees. J Am Board Fam Pract. 1997;10:337-48.
8. Centers for Disease Control. Isolation of *Vibrio cholera* L1 from oysters—Mobile Bay, 1991-1992. MMWR. 1993;42:89-91.
9. Zucker JR. Changing patterns of autochthonous malaria transmission in the United States: a review of recent outbreaks. Emerg Infect Dis. 1996;2:37-43.
10. Centers for Disease Control. Probable locally acquired *Plasmodium vivax* infection transmission—Suffolk County, New York. MMWR. 2000;49:495-8.
11. Patz JA, Epstein PR, Burke TA, Balbus JM. Global climate change and emerging infectious diseases. JAMA. 1996;275:217-23.
12. Shantz PM, Moore AC, Munoz JL, et al. Neurocysticercosis in an orthodox Jewish community in New York City. N Engl J Med. 1992;327:692-5.
13. Cote TR, Convery H, Robinson D, et al. Typhoid fever in the park: epidemiology of an outbreak at a cultural interface. J Community Health.1995:20:451-8.
14. Rodier GR, Ryan MJ, Heymann DL. Global epidemiology of infectious diseases. In: Strickland GT, ed. Hunter's Tropical Medicine, 8th ed. Philadelphia: WB Saunders; 2000:1050.
15. Magill AJ. Fever in the returned traveler. Infect Dis Clin North Am. 1998;12:445-69.
16. Strickland GT. Fever in the returned traveler. Med Clin North Am. 1992;76:1375-92.
17. Doherty JF, Grant AD, Bryceson ADM. Fever as the presenting complaint in travelers returning from the tropics. QJM. 1995;88:277-81.

18. Centers for Disease Control. Imported Dengue—United States, 1997 and 1998. MMWR. 2000;49:248-53.

19. Olliaro P, Cattani J, Wirth D. Malaria, the submerged disease. JAMA. 1996;275:230-3.

20. Centers for Disease Control. Summary of Notifiable Diseases, United States. MMWR. 1998.

21. Humar A, Keystone J. Evaluating fever in travelers returning from tropical countries. BMJ. 1996;312:953-6.

22. Kyriacou DN, Spira AM, Talan DA, Mabey DCW. Emergency department presentation and misdiagnosis of imported falciparum malaria. Ann Emerg Med. 1996;27:696-9.

23. Leder K, Weller P. Malaria. In: Rose BD, ed. UpToDate. 2001;9(1).

24. Paxton LA, Slutsker L, Schultz LJ, et al. Imported malaria in Montagnard refugees settling in North Carolina: implications for prevention and control. Am J Trop Med Hyg. 1996;54:54-7.

25. Bawden MP, Slaten DD, Malone JD. Falciparum malaria in a displaced Haitian population. Trans R Soc Trop Med Hyg. 1995;89:600-3.

26. Diagne N, Rogier C, Sokhna CS, et al. Increased susceptibility to malaria during the early postpartum period. N Engl J Med. 2000;343:598-603.

27. White NJ. Treatment of malaria. N Engl J Med. 1996;335:800-6.

28. Centers for Disease Control. Recommendations for prevention and control of tuberculosis among foreign-born persons. MMWR.1998;47:1-26.

29. Centers for Disease Control. Targeted tuberculin testing and treatment of latent tuberculosis infection. MMWR.2000;49:1-71.

30. Moore M, Onorato IM, McCray E, Castro KG. Trends in drug-resistant tuberculosis in the United States, 1993-1996. JAMA. 1997;278:833-7.

31. Granich R, Zuber PLF, Fussell M, et al. Tuberculosis among foreign-born persons in Southern Florida, 1995. Public Health Rep. 1998;113:552-6.

32. Department of Health and Human Services. Health Information for International Travel, 1999-2000.

33. Li E., Stanley SL. Protozoa. Gastroenterol Clin North Am. 1996;25:471-87.

34. Farthing MJG. Giardiasis. Gastroenterol Clin North Am. 1996;25:493-509.

35. World Health Organization. Hepatitis B Factsheet; 1999.

36. World Health Organization. Weekly Epidemiological Record No. 49; 10 December 1999.

37. Frank C, Mohamed MK, Strickland GT, et al. The role of parenteral anti-schistosomal therapy in the spread of hepatitis C virus in Egypt. Lancet. 2000;355:887.

38. Buchwald D, Lam M, Hooton TM. Prevalence of intestinal parasites and association with symptoms in Southeast Asian refugees. J Clin Pharm Ther. 1995;20:271-5.

39. Salas SD, Heifetz R, Barrett-Connor E. Intestinal parasites in Central American immigrants in the United States. Arch Intern Med. 1990;150:1514-6.

40. Liu LX, Weller PF. Intestinal nematodes. In: Fauci AS, Braunwald E, Isselbacher KJ, et al, eds. Harrison's Principles of Internal Medicine, 14th ed. New York: McGraw-Hill; 1998:1208-12.

41. Gilbert DN, Moellering RC, Sande MA. The Sanford Guide to Antimicrobial Therapy. Vienna, VA: Antimicrobial Therapy; 1999.

42. Muennig P, Pallin D, Sell RL, Man-Suen C. The cost-effectiveness of strategies for the treatment of intestinal parasites in immigrants. N Engl J Med. 1999;340:773-9.

43. Elliott DE. Schistosomiasis. Gastroenterol Clin North Am. 1996;25:599-619.

44. Want P, Adai R. *Helicobacter pylori* in immigrants from East Africa. J Gen Intern Med. 1999;14:567-8.

45. Bardhan PK. Epidemiological features of *Helicobacter pylori* infection in developing countries. Clin Infect Dis. 1997;25:973-8.

46. CDC-NCHSTP-Divisions of HIV/AIDS Prevention. Basic Statistics; 1 December 1998.

47. Tomatis L, Aitio A, Day NE, et al. Cancer: Causes, Occurrence, and Control. IARC Scientific Publications No. 100. WHO International Agency for Research on Cancer; 1990.

48. Gordon NH. Cancer. In: Loue S, ed. Handbook of Immigrant Health. New York: Plenum Press; 1998:389-406.

49. Fendrick AM, Chernew ME, Hirth RA, et al. Clinical and economic effects of population-based *Helicobacter pylori* screening to prevent gastric cancer. Arch Intern Med. 1999;159:142-8.

50. Bosch FX, Ribes J, Borras J. Epidemiology of primary liver cancer. Semin Liver Dis. 1999;19:271-85.

51. Catanzaro A, Moser RJ. Health status of refugees from Vietnam, Laos, and Cambodia. JAMA. 1982;247:1303-8.

52. Anderson JP, Moser RJ. Parasite screening and treatment among Indochinese refugees. JAMA. 1985;253:2229-35.

53. Arfaa F. Intestinal parasites among Indochinese refugees and Mexican immigrants resettled in Contra Costa County, California. J Fam Pract. 1981;12:223-6.

54. Truong DH, Hedemark LL, Mickman JK, et al. Tuberculosis among Tibetan immigrants from India and Nepal in Minnesota, 1992-1995. JAMA. 1997;277:735-8.

55. Barrett-Connor E. Latent and chronic infections imported from Southeast Asia. JAMA. 1978;239:1901-6.

56. Macaw BR, Delay P. Demographics and disease prevalence of two new refugee groups in San Francisco. West J Med. 1985;143:271-5.

57. Massachusetts Department of Public Health. Communicable Disease Update. 1999;7(1).

58. Massachusetts Department of Public Health. Refugees and Immigrants in Massachusetts; 1999.

59. Slutsker L, Tipple M, Keane V, McCance C, Campbell CC. Malaria in East African refugees resettling to the United States: development of strategies to reduce the risk of imported malaria. J Infect Dis. 1995;171:489-93.

60. Arfaa F. Intestinal parasites among Indochinese refugees and Mexican immigrants resettled in Contra Costa County, California. J Fam Pract. 1981;12:223-6.

61. Ciesielski SD, Seed JR, Ortiz JC, Metts J. Intestinal parasites among North Carolina migrant farmworkers. Am J Pub Health. 1992;82:1258-62.

62. Kirchhoff LV. American trypanosomiaisis (Chagas' disease). Gastroenterol Clin North Am. 1996;25:517-29.

63. Ciesielski SD, Seed JR, Esposito DH, Hunter N. The epidemiology of tuberculosis among North Carolina migrant farm workers. JAMA. 1991;265:1715-9.

64. Personal communication. Massachusetts Department of Public Health Statistics. May 1996.

65. Health status of Haitian migrants—U.S. Naval Base, Guantanamo Bay, Cuba—November 1991-April 1992. MMWR. 1993;42:138-40.

66. Bawden MP, Slaten DD, Malone JD. Falciparum malaria in a displaced Haitian population. Trans R Soc Trop Med Hyg. 1995;89:600-3.

67. Rennert G. Implications of Russian immigration on mortality patterns in Israel. Int J Epidemiol. 1994;23:751-6.

68. Guendelman S. Health and disease among Hispanics. In: Loue S, ed. Handbook of Immigrant Health. New York: Plenum Press; 1998:277-301.

69. Takada E, Ford JM, Lloyd LS. Asian Pacific Islander health. In: Loue S, ed. Handbook of Immigrant Health. New York: Plenum Press; 1998:303-27.

70. Faust M, Spilsbury JC, Loue S. African health. In: Loue S, ed. Handbook of Immigrant Health. New York: Plenum Press; 1998:329-48.

71. Preventive Services Task Force. Guide to Clinical and Preventive Services, 2nd ed. Baltimore: Williams & Wilkins; 1996:273.

72. World Health Organization. Web site: www.who.int/vaccines-surveillance/graphics/htmls/hepbprev.htm.

73. World Health Organization. Hepatitis B. Web site: www.who.org/vaccines-diseases/diseases/hepatitis_b.htm.

74. Poland GA. Immunizing the adult immigrant patient: what to do when there are no records. Minn Med. 1995;78:18-20.

75. Centers for Disease Control. Public health dispatch: outbreak of poliomyelitis—Dominican Republic and Haiti, 2000. MMWR. 2000;49:1094-1103.

76. Centers for Disease Control. Recommendations from meeting on strategies for improving global measles control, May 11-12, 2000. MMWR. 2000;49:1116-8.

77. Chen RT, Moses JM, Markowitz LE, Orenstein WA. Adverse events following measles-mumps-rubella and measles vaccinations in college students. Vaccine. 1991;9:297-9.

78. Centers for Disease Control. Rubella among Hispanic adults—Kansas, 1998, and Nebraska, 1999. MMWR. 2000;49:225-8.

79. Munoz N. Prevention of Cancers Associated with Infectious Agents. WHO Publication 9810; 1998.

80. Vento S, Garofano T, Renzini C, et al. Fulminant hepatitis associated with hepatitis A superinfection in patients with chronic hepatitis C. N Engl J Med. 1998;338:286.

81. Bryan JP, Nelson M. Testing for hepatitis A to decrease the cost of hepatitis A prophylaxis with immune globulin or hepatitis A vaccines. Arch Intern Med. 1994;154:663-8.

82. Loue S, Faust M. Intimate partner violence among immigrants. In: Loue S, ed. Handbook of Immigrant Health. New York: Plenum Press; 1998:521-44.

83. Marks G, Garcia M, Solis JM. Health risk behaviors of Hispanics in the United States: findings from HHANES, 1982-84. Am J Public Health. 1990;80:20-6.

84. Castillo R, Waitzkin H, Ramirez Y, Escobar JI. Somatization in primary care, with a focus on immigrants and refugees. Arch Fam Med. 1995;4:637-46.

85. Weinstein JM, Dansky L, Iacopino V. Torture and war trauma survivors in primary care practice. West J Med. 1996;165:112-8.

86. American College of Physicians. The role of the physician and the medical profession in the prevention of international torture and in the treatment of its survivors. Ann Intern Med. 1995;122:607-13.

87. Farmer P. On suffering and structural violence: a view from below. Daedalus. 1996;125:261-83.

88. Fadiman A. The Spirit Catches You and You Fall Down. New York. Farrar, Strauss & Giroux; 1997.

89. Haffner L. Translation is not enough: interpreting in a medical setting. West J Med. 1992;157:255-9.

90. Thamer M, Richard C, Casebeer AW, Ray NF. Health insurance coverage among foreign-born US residents: the impact of race, ethnicity, and length of residence. Am J Pub Health. 1997;87:96-102.

91. Trevino RP, Trevino FM, Medina R, et al. Health care access among Mexican-Americans with different health insurance coverage. J Health Care Poor Underserved. 1996;7:112-21.

92. Siddharthan K, Ahern M. Inpatient utilization by undocumented immigrants without insurance. J Health Care Poor Underserved. 1996;7:355-63.

93. Gany F, Thiel de Bocanegra H. Overcoming the barriers to improving the health of immigrant women. J Am Med Womens Assoc. 1996;51:155-60.

94. Waddell B. United States immigration: a historical perspective. In: Loue S, ed. Handbook of Immigrant Health. New York: Plenum Press; 1998:15.

95. Loue S. Defining the immigrant. In: Loue S, ed. Handbook of Immigrant Health. New York: Plenum Press; 1998:31-6.

96. Federal Register; 26 May 1999.

97. Asch S, Leake B, Gelberg L. Does fear of immigration authorities deter tuberculosis patients from seeking care? West J Med. 1994;161:373-6.

98. Marx JL, Thach AB, Grayson G, et al. The effects of California Proposition 187 on ophthalmology clinic utilization at an inner-city urban hospital. Ophthalmology. 1996;103:847-51.

99. Helman CG. Culture, Health and Illness, 2nd ed. London: Wright; 1990.

100. McPhee SJ. Caring for a 70-year-old Vietnamese woman. JAMA. 2002;287:495-504.

101. Anderson JN. Health and illness in Filipino immigrants. West J Med. 1983;139:811-9.

102. Sontag S. Illness as Metaphor. New York: Vintage; 1978.

103. Perez-Stable EJ, Sabogal F, Otero-Sabogal R, et al. Misconceptions about cancer among Latinos and Anglos. JAMA. 1992;268:3219-23.

104. Chavez LR, Hubbell A, McMullin JM, et al. Understanding knowledge and attitudes about breast cancer. Arch Fam Med. 1995;4:145-50.

105. Kleinman A. Patients and Healers in the Context of Culture. Berkeley: University of California Press; 1980.

106. Surbone A. Truth-telling to the patient. JAMA. 1992;268:1661-2.

107. Carrese JA, Rhodes LA. Western bioethics on the Navajo reservation. JAMA. 1995; 274:826-9.

8

Spirituality and Religion in Health Care

LINDA BARNES, PhD

Insofar as religion is one of the most prevalent and powerful ways in which people find meaning and value in experience, including illness, we physicians would be foolish to ignore the diverse resources for faith that are available to, and being used by, our patients.

D. E. HALL (1)

The world's major religions have long been aware of how prayer and other rituals can answer the spiritual needs of the person who requires physical healing. Since the 1970s, the holistic movement has broadened the definition of health to include not only the body and mind but the spirit and soul (2). This approach has found widespread popular support through various alternative healing practices that have promoted the connection between spirituality and health. In 1998, Eisenberg et al studied the use of complementary and alternative medicine (CAM) by Americans and found the most prevalent therapy to be prayer (3). Eighty-two percent of Americans believe in the healing power of personal prayer, 73% believe that praying for someone can help cure the illness, and 77% believe that God sometimes intervenes to cure people who have a serious illness (4).

Until recently, however, discussion of spirituality and the religious traditions has generally been excluded from the practice of biomedicine. Since the Enlightenment, scientists in Europe and the United States have conceptualized reality as a material universe controlled by fixed physical laws. Science and clinical medicine came to oppose spirit to matter and mind to body. Physicians turned their attention to anatomy, physiology, biochemistry, pathology, and bacteriology. Religious belief and practices were to be separated from scientific knowledge based on empirical data.

Occasionally, however, religion and science meet on common ground, sometimes to collide, sometimes to work together. Legal challenges by the medical community to certain practices of Christian Scientists, Jehovah's Witnesses, and faith healers, particularly in cases involving children, have been well publicized. On the other hand, physicians in their own practices may introduce discussions of spirituality and religion in the face of life-threatening illness and imminent death. Rarely, though, are physicians familiar with the multiple ways that religion and spirituality may shape a patient's sense of health during the course of his or her life.

Yet efforts toward a rapprochement between religion, spirituality, and medicine are gradually emerging. All three represent responses to pain and suffering, leading some authors to point to the broader spiritual dimensions of all health care (5). It has been suggested that the rupture between medicine and spirituality that has characterized biomedicine is an anomaly (6). In addition to the growing popularity of nontraditional ("New Age") workshops and programs on spirituality and healing, mainline religious traditions have expanded healing services.

Because a loosely defined notion of holism has frequently served as the rationale for including spirituality in discussions of patient care, spirituality has routinely been treated as a generic variable, independent of cultural and religious diversity. Caregivers may even openly avoid such diversity, rejecting discussions of religion in favor of spirituality. Few sources addressing spirituality itself locate the topic in relation to cultural competence; few represent religious diversity in relation to cultural diversity; and few examine the interface between religious traditions and related understandings of illness and healing, particularly in connection with cultural versions of religious therapies. Furthermore, as the diversity of the United States has increased in the last decade, the religious affiliations of Americans have diversified (Table 8-1).

Patient Attitudes

According to the World Health Organization, quality of life is composed of six broad domains: 1) physical health, 2) psychological health, 3) level of independence, 4) social relations, 5) environment, and 6) spirituality, religion, and personal beliefs (7). National survey data indicate a significant majority of Americans agree that religion plays an important role in their

Table 8-1 Religious Affiliations in the United States	
Religion	*Percent of Population*
Christianity	76.5
Judaism	1.3
Islam	0.5
Buddhism	0.5
Hinduism	0.4
Unitarian/Universalist	0.3
Wiccan/Pagan/Druid	0.1
Native American (American Indian)	<0.1
Baha'i	<0.1

Source: American Religious Identity Survey, 2001.

experience of life. Ninety-six percent of Americans believe in God, 83% believe that the Bible is the actual or inspired word of God, 75% pray at least once a day, 58% say that "religion is very important in my life," and 43% report having attended worship services within the past week (8).

For many Americans, health and healing are important aspects of their understanding of religious life. For others, the wish to include spirituality in their health care may represent disillusionment with the high-tech, impersonal face of corporate biomedicine. Patients who do not necessarily identify with a particular religious tradition may still view spirituality as a dimension of holistic health and personal growth psychology.

The belief in the strength of the religion and health relationship varies from region to region. A study of 135 family practice patients in Vermont showed 30% of respondents felt that religion generally affected their health and was important in situations such as terminal illness, death, birth, major surgery, general well-being, and major illness. The population comprised mostly married white women, with a mean age of 38.2 years, who reported diverse religious beliefs: Protestant (37%), Catholic (50%), Jewish (1%), other (3%), and none (9%). On the other hand, a cross-sectional survey of 203 family medicine inpatients (120 in Greenville, North Carolina, and 83 in York, Pennsylvania) revealed that 42% had attended a faith-healing service at least once, 94% felt that spiritual health is as important as physical health, 77% said that physicians should consider a patient's spiritual needs, and 37% wanted their physicians to more often discuss religious beliefs. Forty-eight percent wanted their physician to pray with them, and 42%

wanted physicians to ask about faith-healing experiences. However, 68% reported that their physician had never discussed religious beliefs with them, and 12% reported that such discussions had happened only rarely.

Different variables have been identified as predictors of attitudes about prayer and physician involvement in spiritual/religious issues. Frequency of religious service attendance (at least monthly) predicted patient acceptance of physician inquiry into religion and personal faith, as well as acceptance of physician referral to a pastoral professional for spiritual problems (9).

Physician Attitudes

Physician attitudes to their own sense of spirituality, inclusion of religion and spirituality in the patient-doctor relationship, and referral to pastoral professionals have also been studied. Not surprisingly, personal experiences and worldviews related to religion/spirituality and psychotherapy differed sharply between physician members of the American Holistic Medical Association (AHMA) and family practitioners, with AHMA members being more involved than the latter in these issues and related practices (10). Another study found that lack of religious affiliation was common among family medicine faculty and residents in North Carolina and Texas. Physicians were less likely than their patients to pray privately or to hold deeply felt religious beliefs. In part, these findings were explained by age and sex, with the physicians tending to be younger and male, factors often inversely associated with religiosity (11).

In a study involving 146 family physicians and 135 family practice patients in Vermont, Maugans found that patients were more likely than physicians to believe in God (91% vs. 64%), to use prayer (85% vs. 60%), and to feel close to God (74% vs. 43%) (11a). Another study comparing medical students with patients with substance abuse found that the medical students were significantly less religiously and spiritually oriented than patients (12). However, an anonymous survey mailed to a random sample of the American Academy of Family Physicians (physicians involved in direct patient care) indicated that 74% of the physicians attend religious services at least weekly or monthly, 79% report a strong religious or spiritual orientation, and only 4.5% do not believe in God (13). Another study, which examined the nature of work-related stress and coping experienced by African American family physicians in Ohio, indicated that distinctive coping strategies included spirituality (14).

With regard to the inclusion of spirituality and religion in the patient-doctor relationship, a study of 160 Illinois family physicians found that many who believed religion an important influence in the lives of older patients felt it appropriate for the physician to address religious issues. Physicians who believed that religion affects physical or mental health were also more likely to see it as an appropriate topic of discussion (15). Yet Ellis's data show that such physician attitudes do not necessarily translate into actual discussions with patients (15a).

Another study, one involving 180 internal medicine, family, and general practice physicians in the Chesapeake region, found that 33% viewed prayer as a legitimate medical practice; 31% had used it in their own practice; and 53% viewed it as a form of alternative medicine. Additionally, 37% had training in the use of prayer, 49% had knowledge about it, and 72% were interested in receiving training (16). A study of 594 family physicians in seven states showed that 52% were aware of at least one patient who had experienced faith healing. Although 55% agreed that reliance on faith healers often leads to severe medical problems, 44% thought that physicians and faith healers can work together, and 22% believed that faith healers can heal some patients whom physicians cannot help (17).

Ellis found that 86% of the doctors studied felt that inpatients with spiritual questions should be referred to a chaplain (15a). Daaleman and Frey's study of 438 members of the American Academy of Family Physicians reported that more than 80% referred their patients to clergy and pastoral care providers. These cases most frequently involved end-of-life care but also included marital and family counseling, depression, and substance abuse (18).

The Medical Literature: An Overview

Some studies argue more generally that religious involvement is an epidemiologically protective factor (19). Studies correlating religiosity and health outcome have been critiqued because of the difficulty of isolating spirituality and religiosity as significant variables contributing to a specific health outcome (20), questions about the validity of present scientific evidence, conflicting findings, and the lack of evidence in clarity and specificity (21). Some argue that correlation between religious behaviors and health outcomes does not necessarily imply causation (22). There is concern that medical support for the efficacy of faith and prayer may lead some religiously conservative patients, as well as some holistic/New Age patients, to rely on faith, prayer, and visualization to the exclusion of biomedical therapies. Faith can affect health but not always in the way or to the extent that some professionals claim. Also, from the perspective of some religious adherents, the focus on studies based on health outcome may be seen as trivializing religious practice and even as a hubristic testing of divine will. Such studies overlook the larger ideas of healing held by many traditions, in which healing sometimes does not occur until after death. Religion, it is argued, does not need medicine to validate it.

Criteria, Definitions, and Borrowings

The spirituality and religiosity measures used in medical studies attempt to quantify specific aspects of inner, personal experience, individual behaviors, and engagement in a faith community. Some measures such as the Spiritual Well-Being Scale (23) reflect the orientation of specific traditions such as Judaism and Christianity and are therefore not necessarily useful in addressing the broader religious diversity of the United States. Similar questionnaires tend to focus on factors such as religious preference and denominational affiliation; membership in a synagogue or church; belief in God, miracles, life after death, and the literalness of the Bible; and the amount of prayer and Bible reading (8). However, these criteria are not shared by all religious traditions. For example, although immigrants from different countries in Asia are building Buddhist and Hindu shrines and temples throughout the United States, these sites do not tend to have attendance structures of the same kind as synagogues or churches.

Other measures are developed on the unexamined premise that if the variables refer only to *spirituality* and not *religion* (24), they can be assumed to be universally applicable. Although this assumption reflects a common popular perception, it may not adequately reflect the intersecting relationship between the phenomena. It is incorrect to conclude that everyone in American culture means the same thing when using the words *spiritual* or *spirituality*, if these terms are even meaningful in a given cultural context. The increasingly pluralistic racial, ethnic, cultural, and religious landscape of the United States further contributes to the need for a more precise and inclusive understanding of these terms.

Most definitions of *religion* cited in the medical literature are simply not broad enough to capture the diversity of the many religious traditions now present in the United States. Such definitions instead reflect an older scenario in which features of one or two traditions are assumed to be normative and therefore used to define every religious tradition. Also, most definitions of spirituality reflect popular tendencies to polarize religion and spirituality, with religion seen as institutional and spirituality as privatized and personal. Although it is useful to recognize that some people may draw absolute distinctions between religion and spirituality, these two concepts are best understood as highly related, with blurred boundaries in everyday life. The definitions included in this chapter (Boxes 8-1 and 8-2) delineate religious traditions in ways that take into account the findings of recent scholarship and that apply generally to many of the traditions in the United States. These definitions are intended to serve as a reminder of how complex religion and spirituality really are and how often they intersect.

Most of what is referred to as spirituality and spiritual practice refers to some aspect of a particular religious tradition. For example, popularized approaches to meditation in the United States usually derive from Buddhist, Hindu, or Christian practice. For one group of people, this spiritual aspect of its experience may be part of a life-long connection with a particular tradition. Christian spirituality among people of color, for example, tends to be very concrete and deeply rooted in relationships and the community (25).

Even when people identify with a particular tradition, they commonly borrow practices and perspectives from other traditions. Sometimes this borrowing involves the direct appropriation of ideas, practices, and symbols. It happens, for example, when Southern Baptists hold Passover Seders, when self-defined ex-Catholics attend American Indian inspired sweat-lodge workshops, when Jews practice Japanese Zen meditation, or when French Creole practitioners of Vodoun in Louisiana adopt the Virgin of Guadalupe from the Mexican American tradition. Such mixtures are possible, in part, because of globalization, which has led to unprecedented contact between previously distinct traditions; in fact, the phenomenon is worldwide. In the United States, these appropriations and borrowings reflect not only cultural interactions but the freedom to choose one's religious affiliation(s). Mass media intensifies this process, making the curious aware of religious beliefs and practices from around the world.

This degree of contact between groups, along with the possibilities for borrowing and appropriating, can reinforce the claim that spirituality is

---

Box 8-1 Religious Traditions

Religious traditions are expressions of faith in, and reverence for, specific conceptions of ultimate reality. They express one's place in, and relation to, this reality. Ultimate reality may be known as God, Allah, Atman, Nirvana, or by many other names, and is understood and experienced differently by each religious tradition. The forms of faith and reverence of a tradition may be expressed and experienced through

- Sacred stories
- Sacred symbols and objects
- Sacred music, art, and dance
- Devotion—including prayer, meditation, pilgrimage, and other versions of spiritual practice
- Study and interpretation of sacred texts
- Sacred rituals
- Observance of sacred laws
- Reasoned inquiry, or philosophy
- Holy persons—such as saints, prophets, and incarnations of ultimate reality
- Mystical quest, altered states of consciousness, and related disciplines and body-based practices
- Specific approaches to self-cultivation as a profound person
- Ethics and understanding of the proper relationship between self, family, group, earth, and cosmos
- Calls to social transformation, liberation, and justice
- Understanding of what happens after death, and related traditions of dying, death, and memory
- Ongoing relationship with ancestors and the dead
- Relationship with spirits
- Healing

All of these forms are passed down, interpreted, and reinterpreted over time, in different cultural contexts.

---

generic and universal. But when people claim that something is universal, as in the statement, "Down deep, we all share the same spirituality," they may really mean that, "Under the surface, other people's spirituality must be just like mine." Studies assessing stages of diversity awareness show that the assumption of universalism may be used to justify one group's imposing

---

Box 8-2   Spirituality

The term *spirituality* is a way of defining the inner dimension of a religious tradition. It refers to the more private, internal, and individualistic aspects of religious experience. Rather than existing apart from religion, spirituality often refers to the personal experience of practices taken from specific religious traditions (e.g., sacred music, art, and dance, prayer, meditation, mystical quest, altered states of consciousness). Religious traditions and spirituality both address questions of meaning and existential issues as they relate to illness, health, healing, and death.

---

its own values, which may be alien and even offensive, on other groups (26). The assumption that one's own approach is normative also contributes to prejudice formation. Encounters with practices that do not fit under one's own heading of spirituality may result in projecting negative associations with religion onto the worldviews and practices of others. Therefore a more complete understanding of both religion and spirituality is imperative.

An Integrative Model: Religion/Spirituality, Complementary and Alternative Medicine, and Culture

Attempting a Synthesis

Eisenberg et al included prayer as one of 16 versions of CAM (3). However, they did not inquire about the range of other religious therapies associated with the diverse religious traditions in the United States, including those of the mainstream traditions. Nor did the study contain statistically significant estimates of the use of the 16 versions of CAM by African Americans, Hispanic Americans, Asian Americans, or other racial and ethnic groups. Moreover, because the sampling frames were restricted to people who speak English and own telephones, the data were subject to a selection bias. Therefore the practices categorized broadly as CAM more accurately represented those practices favored by predominantly well-educated middle- and upper-middle class European Americans.

A more precise representation of spirituality, religion, and medicine in the United States would examine the intersection of complementary and alternative therapies as specified in Eisenberg's study, the therapies and approaches to healing rooted in the diverse religious traditions of the United States, and the different cultural groups involved (including class differences). The result would show that each of the cultural communities in the United States, including the diverse European American groups, has its preferred approaches to spirituality/religion and related versions of CAM. For example, the majority population's fascination with widely popularized versions of CAM is related to underlying shared beliefs and cultural assumptions tying in with an advocacy of nature, vitalism, science, and spirituality (27). Indeed, for many in this group, healing, spirituality, and CAM intersect.

However, the types of CAM used or recognized by the general population are not necessarily those of other cultural groups. Inclusion of cultural diversity in the scenario helps eliminate the unexamined racial, ethnic, and social class biases of which descriptions of spirituality and CAM are often guilty. It also points more vividly to the plural medical system that now characterizes the United States. In actuality, at no time in the history of the United States has there ever been a unified system of practice. Rather, there has always been a plural system in which different approaches to healing have alternately co-existed and competed. Medical history, however, has often been written as the story of the ascendance of biomedicine, in which other systems of healing have been marginalized and invalidated and have gradually faded out of existence. However, the pervasiveness of a plural approach to healing in the United States has become more visible because of the mainstreaming of majority versions of CAM and because of the growing number of clinician encounters with nonbiomedical practices used by those from different racial and ethnic minority groups.

Characterizing this pluralistic healing landscape is a formidable challenge. For example, Levin and Coreil reviewed over a dozen models of healing, kinds of healers, and medical systems (2). In the end, they acknowledged that none accurately represented the relationship between the parts as now found in the United States. Various terms were partially applicable, such as religious, secular, popular, folk, traditional, marginal, lay, professional, self-care, expert care, scientific, local, regional, and cosmopolitan. However, culturally based religious/spiritual therapies can often be described using most of these terms, making these categories often less than useful.

Classifying Complementary and Alternative Medicine

The National Center for Complementary and Alternative Medicine (NCCAM) at the National Institutes of Health, which defines CAM as health care practices that are not an integral part of conventional medicine (biomedicine), has usefully divided these practices into five major domains: 1) alternative medical systems, 2) body-mind interventions, 3) biologically based treatments, 4) manipulative and body-based methods, and 5) energy therapies (Box 8-3).

Box 8-3   Common Terms Used in Complementary and Alternative Medicine

Alternative medical systems involve theory and practices that have evolved independently of, and often earlier than, conventional biomedical approaches. Many of these traditional systems of medicine exist, including a number of venerable Asian approaches.

Mind-body interventions employ a variety of techniques designed to facilitate the mind's capacity to affect bodily function and symptoms. Not all mind-body interventions are considered complementary or alternative approaches. Many with a well-documented theoretical basis (e.g., patient education, cognitive-behavioral approaches) are now considered mainstream. On the other hand, meditation, certain uses of hypnosis, dance, music, and art therapy, and prayer and mental healing are generally categorized as complementary and alternative approaches.

Biological-based therapies include natural and biologically based practices, interventions, and products, many of which overlap the dietary supplements used in conventional medicine. Included in this category are herbal, special dietary, orthomolecular, and individual biological therapies.

Manipulative and body-based methods include those based on manipulation and movement of the body. For example, chiropractors focus on the relationship between structure (primarily the spine) and function, and how that relationship affects the preservation and restoration of health, whereas massage therapists manipulate the soft tissues of the body in order to normalize them.

Energy therapies focus on affecting the energy fields originating within the body (biofields) or from other sources (electromagnetic fields). Examples include *qi gong, reiki*, and therapeutic touch (see text).

Source: National Center for Complementary and Alternative Medicine.

Note that each of these categories can be examined in light of its specific meaning for each racial and ethnic group and for its intersection with the religious/spiritual traditions and practices of that group.[1]

Alternative Medical Systems

Alternative medical systems are complete systems of theory and practice that have developed independently of, and often previous to, biomedicine. An example is the comprehensive approach to healing that emerged in China based on the experience of the vital force of the body, known as *qi* (pronounced "chee"). Chinese religious and philosophical traditions, as well as Chinese healing methods, share the notion of *qi* as a fundamental property not only of the human system but of all nature and Heaven itself. For a person's *qi* to be out of balance is both to get sick and to be out of step with the events, relationships, and cosmos around oneself. There is no clear dividing line between the two.

Ayurveda is an Indian medical system, one rooted in early Hindu tradition (see Chapter 5). Tibetan medicine, as practiced in a traditional context, cannot be separated from its Buddhist foundations. Likewise, many healing systems brought to the Americas by enslaved Africans retain strong roots in the different native religious traditions out of which they grew. *Santeria,* for example, is an African Cuban religious tradition combining Catholicism with Nigerian tribal beliefs and practices. It includes belief in the magical and healing properties of flowers, herbs, weeds, twigs, and leaves. The American Indian peoples also have their own medicine systems (see Chapter 4).

These alternative medicine systems are generally present in the United States in two forms. The first form occurs in the cultural community of origin, such as the American Indian groups, immigrant communities, and some racial and ethnic minority communities. The second form is an appropriated version of the system, usually found among European Americans. The appropriated version lacks the cultural and religious depth of the original and may be inserted in a fragmented fashion into the realm of New Age spirituality and healing; this version often attracts the notice of the mainstream media. From there, it may be introduced into the biomedical arena, where it is usually separated from its cultural context in all but name, stripped of its religious/spiritual roots, and reduced to a technological intervention.

---

[1] The definitions used here are those of the NCCAM. For further information, see the NCCAM Web site at http://nccamm.nih.gov/nccam/strategic/newleft1.html.

Mind-Body Interventions

Mind-body interventions use different techniques to facilitate the capacity of the mind to affect bodily functions and symptoms. Of the examples listed by NCCAM, many, such as meditation, certain uses of hypnosis, dance, music, prayer, and mental healing, intersect with different religious and spiritual systems. In some cases, these examples represent specific practices of the alternative medical systems discussed above. In others, they may be specific practices appropriated and revised for a European American audience.

Healing practices of the mainstream religious traditions, with all their cultural variations, also fall under the heading of mind-body interventions, such as the use of prayer, healing services, ritual processions for saints, pilgrimages, witnessing an icon to which healing properties are attributed, and exorcism. The trance possession states of Vodoun and Santeria, the sacred music and dance of American Indians, and Buddhist and Hindu versions of meditation are examples of other culturally and religiously/spiritually based mind-body interventions. When appropriated by a majority audience, these practices are frequently represented as the mystical aspects of the religious traditions of origin.

Biologically Based Therapies

Biologically based therapies include natural and biologically based practices, interventions, and products, many of which overlap with the use of dietary supplements by conventional medicine. Included are herbal, special dietary, orthomolecular, and individual biological therapies. Some of these therapies may represent specific aspects of alternative medical systems, where the use of an herb or a combination of herbs may simultaneously have ritual/sacred meaning as well as physiological meaning. Both aspects may be assumed to be necessary for healing to take place. Herbs sold in health food stores may be associated with energy, which can overlap with Americanized ideas about *qi* and with understandings of spirituality traceable to a New Age orientation.

Manipulative and Body-Based Methods and Energy Therapies

Manipulative and body-based methods are based on manipulation and movement of the body, such as chiropractic and massage. Energy therapies focus on energy fields originating within the body (biofields) or from other sources (electromagnetic fields). Some forms of energy therapy attempt to control these biofields by applying pressure and manipulating the body by placing one's hands in or through the fields. NCCAM differentiates between body-based methods and energy therapies on the basis of the intention of the energy therapies to affect an energy field. In reality, the distinction is not always entirely evident, insofar as some chiropractors and practitioners of massage think of their treatments as influencing the patient's energy. One should note that the existence of these energy fields has not been proven experimentally.

Three examples of energy therapy can be discussed briefly. *Qi gong* is a component of traditional Chinese medicine that combines movement, meditation, and regulation of breathing to enhance the flow of vital energy (*qi*) in the body, to improve blood circulation, and to enhance immune function. Some acupuncturists practice *qi gong* to become more sensitive to the flow of *qi* in themselves and their patients. *Reiki* (Japanese for "universal life energy") is based on the belief that by channeling spiritual energy through the practitioner the spirit is healed, which in turn heals the body. Therapeutic touch, a third kind of energy therapy, derives from the ancient technique of "laying-on of hands" and is based on the premise that the healing force of the therapist affects the patient's recovery and that healing is promoted when the body's energies are in balance.

Thus, in some respects, the energy therapies represent the intersection of mind-body and body-based therapies. Because these methods involve the cultivation of meditative states, they may form part of the user's religious/spiritual practice.

These five domains illustrate the fluid boundaries between categories of culture, CAM, and spirituality and religion. They serve as a reminder that when nonbiomedical therapies enter the picture they usually go hand-in-hand with the cultural orientation of the patient and may be an expression of his or her spiritual/religious worldview. For this reason, the use of such therapies may be important to the patient according to what he or she holds most sacred.

Beliefs and Attitudes

The concept of *health* varies depending on a person's religious/spiritual worldview and is necessarily related to one's understanding of ultimate human possibility. Such possibility may be described as salvation, awakening or enlightenment, nirvana, being venerated as an ancestor, having a share in the world to come or in paradise, and many other formulations. The meaning and importance of one's health during life may therefore be secondary to an ultimate healing that may take place after death.

Likewise, each worldview has its own way of explaining why people suffer. Sometimes the explanation takes the form of stories. Sometimes suffering is considered a test, or a punishment, or even a blessing. None of these explanations can be fully separated from the larger issue of attempting to explain and address suffering, which is a meeting ground for medicine, religion, and spirituality.

It is common belief in the United States that a person comprises a body, mind, and soul or spirit, yet this conceptualization is not universal. Different religious/spiritual traditions envision the person in different ways. *Qi*-based systems think of the person as nothing but *qi,* organized in different patterns of density, with palpable channels of *qi* flowing through the system as a whole. In traditional Chinese thought, a person had as many as eleven souls. After death, some of these souls took on a more ethereal dimension and located themselves in the ancestor tablets; others were denser and were buried with the body. If not acknowledged with periodic offerings, they might inflict illness and misfortune as hungry ghosts.

Knowing how the person is conceptualized in the patient's religious tradition can provide the clinician with a better understanding of what an individual patient is likely to feel about his or her illness. Because beliefs about sickness and health relate to the concept of person, the physician's choice of therapeutic options may be circumscribed. One cannot, however, assume that all individuals from a particular cultural group share the same views.

Physicians may assume that religious or spiritual issues are, for the most part, pertinent in cases of life-threatening illness and end-of-life care. However, basic ideas of good health and healthy living may also be predicated on the importance of spirituality. The very food one does or does not eat, as well as what one does or does not drink, may be prescribed or proscribed by one's religious tradition (28).

Clinicians are sometimes encouraged to promote specific ideas of healthy sexuality. However, the assumption of a normative ideal of healthy sexuality overlooks the degree to which different religions have different teachings about what is considered to be sexual morality. Liberal and conservative interpretations of a traditional teaching are also important factors. Gender identity may be strongly shaped by religious teachings about the identities of men and women and their relationship to one another, but in some instances religion and culture overlap in an attempt to legitimize the dominance of men over women (29). Religion and culture may also converge in "sanctioning" prejudice, hatred, violence, homophobia, and even hate crimes.

Attitudes toward family planning and birth control are sometimes informed by religious teachings. Higher levels of fertility have been associated with religious prohibitions on birth control and with the promotion of childbearing and traditional family and gender roles (30). A study conducted in the Dominican Republic, Egypt, Indonesia, and Thailand on the acceptability of Norplant contraceptive implants revealed that one of the three leading factors influencing acceptability were cultural and religious variables (31). A study of Vietnamese refugee women's attitudes about family planning revealed that cultural and religious beliefs directed the women's choice of method (32). Religion and culture can also influence attitudes toward genetic counseling (33) and abortion.

Religion may be the most significant determinant of family planning and birth control practices, but income, literacy, and urbanization are important factors also (34). One study hypothesized that the religiosity and spirituality of Mexican American women may function as one of the factors protecting them and their infants through the prenatal and antenatal phases of life, based on data showing that Mexican American women of relatively lower socioeconomic status deliver significantly fewer low birth weight babies and lose fewer babies to all causes during infancy than do women of other racial/ethnic groups (35). Increased family support, back migration, and the absence of negative health effects of acculturation are also important. Spirituality may serve as a stress moderator (36); high levels of spiritual well-being and church attendance allow low-income Hispanic women to deal with the stress of poverty, for example (37).

Patients may also interpret specific health conditions in religious or spiritual terms. For example, a study of the under-use of screening services and early treatment centers by non-Mexican-American Hispanic adults with diabetes showed that 78% of the 104 adults surveyed (most of whom were women) believed they had diabetes because it was God's will (38). Resort to biomedical therapies may be perceived as indicating a lack of faith and treatment may be refused. On the other hand, the patient may view the clinician as help provided by God and may see turning to biomedical therapies as trusting in God to provide the care one needs.

Religiosity can have both positive and negative effects on the etiology and treatment of mental illness. Traditions that emphasize guilt can contribute to low self-esteem and other mental and emotional problems. But religion can also serve as a cultural strength to help manage the course of mental illness (39). In some cases, a system of religious therapies may serve as the patient's way of coping with and healing mental illness. One qualitative study that compared the attitudes of black and white patients with depression and of physicians and social workers regarding help-seeking behavior showed that black patients raised more concerns about spirituality and stigma than white patients did. Patients made more comments than professionals concerning the impact of spirituality as one of the factors related to their help-seeking behavior and adherence to treatment (40).

Another area where intersections of religion/spirituality, culture, and diverse approaches to healing occur is in relation to alcohol and substance abuse. One study suggests that religious attendance correlates negatively with alcohol use (41). One of the most widely publicized programs related to addressing alcohol abuse, Alcoholics Anonymous (AA), presents itself as a spiritual program of recovery. The first wave of diffusion brought AA to the predominantly Anglo-Saxon and Protestant world. The second wave reached the broader Americas and the European Catholic countries. More recent connections have been established with newly industrialized nations.

However, Alcoholics Anonymous remains largely a phenomenon of wealthy, industrialized countries. Moreover, the underlying structure of the understanding of spirituality is Protestant Christianity. The program has encountered cultural points of resistance related to its advocacy of a "surrender" to a Higher Power, which may be experienced as the promotion of powerlessness, an issue for groups contending with concerns about low self-esteem, dysfunctional family structure, communication difficulties, and institutionalized and internalized racism. Therefore even programs ostensibly based on a one-size-fits-all version of spirituality face challenges related to multiculturalism. Alternative approaches have drawn on conceptual frameworks related to core African-centered beliefs (42) or on symbolic healing resources rooted in North American Indian versions of spirituality (43).

Perceptions of persisting conditions such as disability have been shaped by scientific and religious traditions. The medical model of disability and the emerging genetic model influence the way ideas of disability are constructed and how we treat people with disability. In some cases, religious traditions have contributed to views that the disabled person is in some way being tested or punished and that he or she is the object of pity or charity. However, spiritual and religious factors can also enable individuals with disability and chronic illness to cope successfully by providing inner resources and strengths. One study argues that religion and spirituality may be underused resources in the rehabilitation process and in the ongoing lives of persons with disabilities (44).

Religiousness has also been associated with coping with cancer. One study of 290 women with familial breast cancer showed that among women who perceived themselves to be at low risk of developing breast cancer, those with higher levels of spiritual faith were significantly less likely to go for testing for alterations in the *BRCA1* and *BRCA2* genes (44a). However, among women with high levels of perceived risk, rates of test use were high, regardless of spiritual faith. A study of 25 Hispanic women and 25 Anglo-American women diagnosed with breast cancer showed that the Hispanic women scored higher on intrinsic religiousness and consequently total religious well-being, whereas for Anglo-American women intrinsic religiousness was a strong predictor of spiritual well-being and hopefulness. The study concluded that while religiosity may be an important factor in the psychological and spiritual health of women with breast cancer, cultural differences may also shape the specific nature of the influence of religiosity (45). A study of how Mexican and Central American patients manage cancer pain showed that culture, family beliefs, and religion contribute significantly to its expression and management (46).

Moreover, as one study of Egyptian American oncology patients suggests, dietary restrictions, social conduct, and religious observances are among the areas that require understanding on the part of the clinical staff (47). Fuller knowledge of the patient's condition may be gained by an interpretation provided by a religiously based system of healing, as in one case of cancer interpreted within an Ayurvedic framework (48).

A patient's religious orientation, as well as that of family members, may influence patient experience of anesthesia, surgery, and post-operative pain. For example, one study suggests that privacy and modesty, family roles, body language, group decision making, communication distances, and folk beliefs are important factors among Arab Muslim patients. More broadly speaking, care of Muslim patients requires a familiarity with the central relationship between religion and family and the influence of religion and family on health care in general (see Chapter 6) (49).

Attitudes toward aging may also be influenced by religion and spirituality, particularly in regard to a person's understanding of what happens after death. One study indicated that persons with lower death depression had greater strength of conviction, stronger belief in the afterlife, and were less likely to say that the most important aspect of religion is that it offers the possibility of life after death (50). Another study showed stronger religious beliefs were associated with a lower tolerance of suicide. Personal religious beliefs and, for men, exposure to a religious environment may protect against suicide by reducing its acceptability (51). Although religions differ on the meaning of death and what takes place after death, few of them view death pessimistically (52). Not only have many of these traditions formulated varying positions on end-of-life decisions, autopsy, organ donation, and subsequent treatment of the body but individuals and families from different cultural groups have their own interpretations of these topics. Grief may also be influenced by culturally based spiritual and religious views of death and loss.

Additionally, the troubled history of biomedicine and some racial and ethnic groups has been chronicled and challenged within religious frameworks (53). Theologians can represent the perspective of some of those most deeply afflicted by systemic biases. They point to ways in which religiosity, in its communal forms, can offer a healing response to health problems and excess deaths resulting from the oppressive social structures of racism, sexism, and classism, and related forms of violence. In particular, African American womanist theologians have promoted an integrated understanding of life and health in relation to the internal psychological constructions of African American womanhood. They have also argued for a therapeutic Black church and womanist communities of care and support (26,54).

A Physician's Guide to Addressing Spiritual and Religious Issues

For physicians to address the topic of culture, spirituality, religion, and healing, two sets of skills are indispensable. The first involves the cultivation of self-awareness and reflection on the components of one's own identity. These factors are present in every clinical encounter and influence how one hears what patients have to say. The second involves learning strategies for talking with patients about the topic and for responding to what they say.

Knowing One's Identity

Many efforts to train culturally competent clinicians focus on promoting knowledge about other cultural groups without necessarily teaching clinicians to be attuned to their own perceptions of, and responses to, difference. Learning about cultural groups and social classes other than one's own is important, but without a certain kind of self-awareness the physician may project and act out biases. Disciplines such as family therapy have come to recognize that cultural sensitivity involves exploring personal cultural issues, including orientation to religion, spirituality, and related approaches to healing.

One important tool for building awareness of personal cultural identity and its implications for interactions with people from different cultures is the cultural genogram, an extended family tree in which one identifies multiple dimensions of difference and cultural formation in order to learn where and how one may have internalized different kinds of bias (55). These cultural variables can be focused through the lens of one's own religious/spiritual formation and identity (Box 8-4). A growing body of literature indicates

---

Box 8-4   Spirituality/Religion Self-Assessment Questions

1. Did any member of your family immigrate to the United States for religious reasons?
2. If other than American Indian, under what conditions did your family/ancestors enter the United States (immigrant, political refugee, slave, etc.)?
3. What were/are your group's experiences with oppression? Did any of this have to do with religious reasons? (Group can refer to racial/cultural/religious/ethnic identity.)
4. Map the religious background(s) of the different members in your genogram.
5. Did these religious identities stay the same? If not, why?
6. Is there a dominant religious tradition in your family tree? If so, what is it?
7. Are there minority orientations in your family (e.g., someone who may have decided to define themselves differently)? If so, what has been the effect on the larger family?
8. If there was more than one religious tradition in your family, how were the differences negotiated? What were the intergenerational consequences? How has this had an impact on you personally?

(Cont'd.)

Box 8-4 (continued)

9. Do you come from a religious background that taught you values about work? About success? About poverty? If so, in what ways? Were there different messages from different branches of your family? How did these influences affect your understanding of social class (including your own and others)?

10. Do you come from a religious background that taught you values about gender (i.e., men's and women's role identities)? If so, in what ways?

11. Do you come from a religious background in which your group had prejudices or stereotypes about itself? Did this affect you? If so, how?

12. What prejudices or stereotypes do other groups have about your group? Did this affect you? If so, how?

13. What prejudices or stereotypes does your group have about other groups? Did this affect you? If so, how?

14. Do you come from a religious background that thought about family in particular ways? If so, how?

15. Do you come from a religious background that included practices related to healing? If so, in what ways?

16. Do you come from a religious background that shaped your understanding about being sick? About pain? About suffering? If so, how?

17. Do you come from a religious background that influenced your thinking about being a biomedical caregiver?

18. Do you come from a religious background that shaped your thoughts about healing? If so, in what ways?

19. Have you:
    a) continued to be part of a tradition from your upbringing?
    b) rejected a tradition of your upbringing?
    c) changed your relationship in other ways with a tradition of your upbringing?
    d) converted to another tradition?
    e) composed your own private version of spirituality based on pieces drawn from different traditions?

20. Have you adopted other versions of spiritual/religious practice and thinking into your own worldview? If so, in what ways?

21. Depending on your relationship with your family history as pertains to religious background, have you found yourself trying to change your understanding of any of the topics above? If so, in what ways?

Adapted from Hardy KV, Laszloffy TA. The cultural genogram: key to training culturally competent family therapists. J Marital Fam Ther. 1995:21:227-37.

that the beliefs and values a physician brings to clinical care are crucial to effective functioning (Case 8-1) (55).

Talking to the Patient

Strategies

In a plural medical system, patients routinely create a composite health care matrix in which the physician is only one part. Physicians are often unaware that a patient may rely on other approaches to healing besides the biomedical. Too often, also, physicians do not realize the extent to which strongly held religious and spiritual beliefs may influence a patient's willingness or eagerness to follow prescribed treatment and therapy.

Virtually all spiritual/religious traditions have a place for the physician/healer and the practice of healing. Examples are provided by sources on Judaism (56), Christianity (57), Islam (58), Hinduism (59), Buddhism (60), Navajo (61), Hmong shamanism (62), and African-derived traditions (63). There are also anthologies of introductory overviews (64,65) and a number of useful Web sites.[2] The primary limitation of many of these sources is that they do not address the diversity *within* traditions, or the intracultural variations. For example, Italian, Irish, Chicano, Vietnamese, and Indian versions of Roman Catholicism have underlying commonalities yet significantly diverge from each other. Therefore a general understanding of a tradition and how it views the relation between the believer and illness can only be a preliminary step to full physician-patient communication.

A patient's spirituality may be governed almost entirely by cultural norms, in opposition to cultural norms, or by a combination of cultural norms and individual life experience (66). Variations will also present themselves within families (degree of acculturation) and between generations. Whether a patient adheres to the religious/spiritual ways of his or her family, has converted to another tradition, or has simply rejected the family's religious/spiritual beliefs is another factor that may come into play when critical health decisions need to be made.

There are many approaches to inquiring about the importance of religious and spiritual beliefs as they relate to health care. For example, a task force of the American College of Physicians-American Society of Internal

---

[2] For Web sites on different religious traditions, see http://www.ciolek.com/WWWVLPages/BuddhPages/OtherRelig.html, http://www.religioustolerance.org, and http://www.lib.iun.indiana.edu/trannurs.htm.

CASE 8-1   A 47-YEAR-OLD JEHOVAH'S WITNESS WHO REFUSES A BLOOD TRANSFUSION

Mr Robinson, a 47-year-old African American who works as an insurance adjuster, is a practicing Jehovah's Witness. He has made clear to his primary care physician his desire, based on his beliefs, not to receive blood products. Mr Robinson, a former smoker, has hypertension and high cholesterol.

Mr Robinson presents to the emergency department with light-headedness after 2 days of passing melena. His blood pressure is 100/60 with a pulse of 116 with postural changes. An NG tube passed into his stomach reveals heme + coffee grounds appearing material. Rectal examination reveals grossly heme + black stool. Hematocrit is 28 on presentation and decreases to 22 after Mr Robinson receives some intravenous fluids. The emergency department physician, who has been unable to reach Mr Robinson's primary care physician, orders a blood transfusion, which Mr Robinson refuses, saying his religion forbids it. When the physician persists, Mr Robinson becomes angry. When a psychiatrist appears to assess his competency, Mr Robinson threatens to leave the hospital.

DISCUSSION

Physicians face a special challenge when treating Jehovah's Witnesses. Members of this faith have deep religious convictions against accepting homologous or autologous whole blood, packed red blood cells, white blood cells, or platelets. There are more than half a million Jehovah's Witnesses in the United States who do not accept blood transfusions. Courts have ruled definitively that individuals can refuse even lifesaving interventions and that they must give informed consent before being treated with blood transfusions.

In Mr Robinson's case the emergency room physician was obligated to explain the benefits of transfusion and the risks of declining such treatment, then to follow the patient's wishes. It is inappropriate to obtain a psychiatric consultation to assess competency unless there are clear signs of incompetence. Refusing blood, even in this circumstance, does not constitute incompetence; here, the request for psychiatric consultation likely reflects the physician's own bias against the beliefs held by the patient.

Medicine has suggested four basic questions in relation to palliative care (Box 8-5) (67). If the patient indicates that religious factors influence his or her understanding of illness and treatment, the physician may decide to support this orientation. Support, in this case, simply means acknowledging and respecting the patient's religious orientation. If the patient does not find such views important, it is not appropriate to pursue the topic. If a religious or spiritual orientation is in conflict with what the physician judges to be a necessary biomedical therapy, the physician should provide the patient with information that will allow them to work together toward a compromise (Case 8-2).

There are diagnostic tools with which to assess spiritual distress (68). There are also tools for taking a spiritual history (11a), for identifying spiritual issues (69), and for discussing what one study defines as "wellness spirituality" for older adults (70). The primary limitation of most of these tools is that they pertain most directly to patients with a Christian orientation and may not be useful in other traditions. It is important to discuss these tools with the religious leaders in one's location in order to modify them for the patient population being treated.

In 1990 the Committee on Religion and Psychiatry of the American Psychiatric Association issued a Position Statement entitled "Guidelines Regarding Possible Conflict Between Psychiatrists' Religious Commitments and Psychiatric Practice." These guidelines emphasize the importance of respecting differences between the religious/spiritual orientations of the clinician and patient (71). Also, the fourth edition of the Diagnostic and Statistical Manual of Mental Disorders (DSM-IV) now includes a diagnostic category for "religious or spiritual problems" under the section "Other

---

Box 8-5   Questions for Exploring Religion and Spirituality in Palliative Care

• Is faith (religion, spirituality) important to you at this time?
• Has faith (religion, spirituality) been important to you at other times in your life?
• Do you have someone to talk to about religious matters?
• Would you like to discuss religious matters with someone?

Adapted from Lo B, Quill T, Tulsky J. Discussing palliative care with patients. Ann Intern Med. 1999;130:744-9.

CASE 8-2   A 76-YEAR-OLD WOMAN WHO REFUSES CANCER TREATMENT ON RELIGIOUS GROUNDS

Mrs A— is a 76-year-old Somali woman who is diagnosed with breast cancer that is metastatic to her bones. After a long discussion with her physician about various options, including surgical resection, radiation therapy, and chemotherapy, she states that she does not want treatment. She says, "My life is determined by God. If it is God's will that I die now, then I will not question it." Mrs A— explains that she believes God determines her destiny and that it is wrong to question or challenge it. Her doctor asks her about the importance of faith in her life. She replies that she is very religious and is not afraid to die. Her doctor respects her decision and asks whether there is anything he can do for her. She reveals that she is afraid she will have a lot of pain. She and her physician agree upon a plan that will allow her to get the help she desires if her pain becomes worse.

DISCUSSION

It can be difficult for a physician to accept a patient's decision to refuse treatment, particularly insofar as the doctor's role is usually defined in relation to providing therapeutic interventions. It is useful to remember that healing may mean additional things to the patient. Given Mrs A—'s faith structure, for example, it is likely that she does not view her life as ending with her physical death. In cases of life-threatening or terminal illness, it can be important to understand not only how the patient interprets the illness itself, but also how he or she views what happens after death. Most religious traditions see death as a transition into some other state of being, sometimes conceptualized as an ultimate form of healing. In this case, by asking Mrs A— whether she would like anything else done, the patient is given the occasion to define what she needs, which can be experienced as deeply healing.

Conditions That May Be a Focus of Clinical Attention." With this category, DSM-IV attempts to present these topics in ways that will enhance cultural sensitivity rather than pathologize religion and spirituality. Definitions, types, and clinical significance of religious and spiritual problems have been clarified (72).

Kleinman proposes that one begin by asking the patient about his or her understanding of the illness under consideration (73). For example: "What do you think caused your illness? What kind of treatment do you think you need? What do you most fear? How has the illness affected you and your family?" Family members should be asked similar questions. The responses may lead the physician into the areas of religiosity and possible spiritual crisis.

In some cases, these issues may not be explicitly stated at first. Therefore, the broader skill, as in all effective medical care, involves developing the capacity to listen in a way that is personally respectful, clinically insightful, and aimed at understanding rather than agreement or disagreement. It may also be important to ask, and listen openly, about the things the patient and family have done to treat the problem, including religious/spiritual therapies and support. This process does not need to be complicated. One of the author's colleagues has found it extremely helpful in his clinical practice simply to ask, "What do we need to do to heal the whole person?" From there, one may want to explore with the patient the possibility of a consultation with, and a referral to, a spiritual/religious caregiver. It may be helpful to build an ongoing relationship with available chaplaincy services and local consultants in different traditions. One can also refer to a patient-preferred spiritual care provider.

In general, it is wise to assume that patients may have religious and spiritual concerns about their illness and that the illness itself may be experienced as a spiritual crisis. If asked, patients are often willing to explain what these concerns are, how they fit into a broader religious/spiritual worldview, and how related therapies are conceptualized and used.

Barriers and Criticism

One study has indicated that barriers to discussing spiritual issues with patients include lack of time, lack of training in how to obtain a spiritual history, difficulty identifying patients who want to discuss spiritual issues, and concerns about projecting beliefs onto patients (15a). Physicians, uncomfortable with this subject, can also be uncertain about how to manage spiritual issues raised by patients and may feel that spiritual issues should take a lower priority than medical issues. In contrast to data cited earlier showing that many physicians felt it was appropriate to address religious issues, this study showed that approximately one third of physicians felt that expressing spiritual concerns was not appropriate to the physician's role, believed that patients do not want to share spiritual concerns with their physicians, worried about the effects of a lack of continuity with their patients, and found it difficult to know how to use appropriately understood language in discussion of spiritual issues.

Similar concerns are raised by those opposed to the discussion of spiritual issues in the physician's office. They argue that physicians lack appropriate training in this area and step outside their domain if they query patients about religious beliefs and give advice on spiritual matters. Physicians, in short, are unqualified to offer guidance on matters of faith. For this reason, critics suggest, the inclusion of such topics may lead to the abuse of a physician's authority, particularly when a patient is emotionally and physically vulnerable. Patients may be made to feel guilty or not faithful enough if they were instructed to pray, did so, and did not get better. In short, it is argued, medicine should not take on religious practices as adjunctive treatments. Moreover, the cultural and religious diversity now found in many patient populations is a challenge even to hospital chaplains, who are trained as religious/spiritual counselors. Physicians, it is argued, are not prepared to enter into discussions with patients whose religious/spiritual beliefs may differ from their own. Although critics agree that religion/spirituality may serve as an important resource in helping patients cope, they argue that these topics should not be singled out but rather subsumed under more general questions about coping strategies (74).

Many barriers do exist and critics often make salient points. Nonetheless, it is important to ascertain whether spiritual/religious issues inform a patient's understanding of health care. Such issues have implications for treatment options and therefore influence medical outcomes. Despite arguments that spiritually involved and informed physicians are bypassing or even usurping the role of religious counselors (75), many physicians consider such inquiry a necessary precursor to making appropriate referrals to trained religious figures or to seeking such assistance themselves when treatment compromises are necessary on religious grounds.

Summary

The influence and importance of psychological and social factors in relation to bodily processes have become well recognized. Such factors transform the biological event of a disease into the subjective experience of illness. Culturally based understandings of religion, spirituality, and healing are important components of patient reaction to illness and disease. Moreover, these beliefs may determine which biomedical therapies the patient is willing to accept. Particularly when the issue is one of suffering and, perhaps, spiritual crisis, it is worth discovering what the patient will say when asked, "What do we need to do to heal the whole person?"

REFERENCES

1. Hall DE. Medicine and religion. N Engl J Med. 2000;343:1340-1.
2. Levin JS, Coreil J. "New Age" healing in the United States. Soc Sci Med. 1986;23:889-97.
3. Eisenberg DM, Davis RB, Ettner SL, et al. Trends in alternative medicine use in the United States, 1990-1997: results of a follow-up national survey. JAMA. 1998;280:1569-75.
4. Yankelovich Partners. Telephone poll for Time/CNN, June 12-13, 1996. Time. 1996; Jun 24;58-62.
5. Schwartz SG. Holistic health: seeking a link between medicine and metaphysics. JAMA. 1991;266:3064.
6. Sulmasy DP. Is medicine a spiritual practice? Acad Med. 1999;74:1002-5.
7. World Health Organization. The structure of the WHOQOL-100. Available at http://www.who.int/msa/mnh/mhp/ql5.htm.
8. Gallup G Jr, Lindsay DM. Surveying the Religious Landscape: Trends in U.S. Beliefs. Harrisburg, PA: Morehouse Publishing; 1999.
9. Daaleman TP, Nease DE Jr. Patient attitudes regarding physician inquiry into spiritual and religious issues. J Fam Pract. 1994;39:564-8.
10. Goldstein MS, Sutherland C, Jaffe DT, Wilson J. Holistic practitioners and family practitioners: similarities, differences and implications for health policy. Soc Sci Med. 1988; 26:853-61.
11. Oyama O, Koenig HG. Religious beliefs and practices in family medicine. Arch Fam Med. 1998;7:431-5.
11a. Maugans TA. The spiritual history. Arch Fam Med. 1996;5:11-16.
12. Goldfarb LM, Galanter M, McDowell D, et al. Medical student and patient attitudes toward religion and spirituality in the recovery process. Am J Drug Alcohol Abuse. 1996;22:549-61.
13. Daaleman TP, Frey B. Spiritual and religious beliefs and practices of family physicians: a national survey. J Fam Pract. 1999;48:98-104.
14. Post DM, Weddington WH. Stress and coping of the African-American physician. J Nat Med Assoc. 2000;92:70-5.
15. Koenig HG, Bearon LB, Dayringer R. Physician perspectives on the role of religion in the physician-older patient relationship. J Fam Pract. 1989;28:441-8.

15a. Ellis MR, Vinson DC, Ewigman B. Addressing spiritual concerns of patients: family physicians' attitudes and practices. J Fam Pract. 1999;48:105-9.

16. Berman BM, Singh BK, Lao L, et al. Physicians' attitudes toward complementary or alternative medicine: a regional survey. J Am Board Fam Pract. 1995;8:361-6.

17. King DE, Sobal J, Haggerty J 3rd, et al. Experiences and attitudes about faith healing among family physicians. J Fam Pract. 1992;35:158-62.

18. Daaleman TP, Frey B. Prevalence and patterns of physician referral to clergy and pastoral care providers. Arch Fam Med. 1998;7:548-53.

19. Matthews DA, McCullough ME, Larson DB, et al. Religious commitment and health status: a review of the research and implications for family medicine. Arch Fam Med. 1998;7:118-24.

20. Daaleman TP, Frey B. Association between spirituality and health hard to measure [Letter, Comment]. Fam Med. 1998;30:470-1.

21. Sloan RP, Bagiella E, Powell T. Religion, spirituality, and medicine. Lancet. 1999;353:664-7.

22. Sloan RP, VandeCreek L. Religion and medicine: why faith should not be mixed with science. Available on several Web sites including Medscape.

23. Ellison CW, Paloutzian RF. The Spiritual Well-Being Scale. Nyack, NY: Life Advance; 1982.

24. Hatch RL, Burg MA, Naberhaus DS, Helmich LK. The spiritual involvement and beliefs scale: development and testing of a new instrument. J Fam Pract. 1998;46:476-86.

25. Musgrove CF, Allen CE, Allen CJ. Spirituality and the health of women of color. Am J Public Health. 2002;92:557-60.

26. Llerena-Quinn R. How do assumptions of difference and power affect how and what we teach? AFTA Newsletter. 2001;82:22-6.

27. Kaptchuk TJ, Eisenberg DM. The persuasive appeal of alternative medicine. Ann Int Med. 1998;129:1061-5.

28. Shatenstein B, Ghadirian P. Influences on diet, health behaviors and their outcome in select ethno-cultural and religious groups. Nutrition. 1998;14:223-30.

29. LaChat MR. Religion's support for the domination of women: breaking the cycle. Nurse Pract. 1988;13:31-4.

30. Schenker JG, Rabenou V. Family planning: cultural and religious aspects. Hum Reprod. 1993;8:969-76.

31. Zimmerman M, Haffey J, Crane E, et al. Assessing the acceptability of Norplant implants in four countries: findings from focus group research. Stud Fam Plann. 1990;21:92-103.

32. Kuss T. Family planning experiences of Vietnamese women. J Community Health Nurs. 1997;14:155-68.

33. Swinford AE, el-Fouly MH. Islamic religion and culture: principles and implications for genetic counseling. Birth Defects: Original Article Series. 1987;23:253-7.

34. Pick JB, Tellis GL, Butler EW. Fertility determinants in the oil region of Mexico. Soc Biol. 1989;36:45-66.

35. Magana A, Clark NM. Examining a paradox: does religiosity contribute to positive birth outcomes in Mexican American populations? Health Educ Q. 1995;22:96-109.

36. Bjorck JP, Lee YS, Cohen LH. Control beliefs and faith as stress moderators for Korean American versus Caucasian American Protestants. Am J Community Psychol. 1997;25:61-72.

37. Rojas DZ. Spiritual well-being and its influence on the health of Hispanic women. In: Torres S, ed. Hispanic voices: Hispanic health educators speak out. New York: NLN Press; 1996:213-29.

38. Zaldivar A, Smolowitz J. Perceptions of the importance placed on religion and folk medicine by non-Mexican-American Hispanic adults with diabetes. Diabetes Educator. 1994;20:303-6.

39. Leffley HP. Culture and chronic mental illness. Hosp Comm Psych. 1990;41:277-86.

40. Cooper-Patrick L, Powe NR, Jenckes MW, et al. Identification of patient attitudes and preferences regarding treatment of depression. J Gen Intern Med. 1997;12:431-8.

41. Maes HH, Neale MC, Martin NG, et al. Religious attendance and frequency of alcohol use. Twin Research. 1999;2:169-79.

42. Rowe D, Grills C. African-centered drug treatment: an alternative conceptual paradigm for drug counseling with African-American clients. J Psychoactive Drugs. 1993;25:21-33.

43. Waldram JB. Aboriginal spirituality: symbolic healing in Canadian prisons. Cult Med Psychiatry. 1993;17:345-62.

44. Underwood-Gordon L, Peters DJ, Bijur P, Fuhrer M. Roles of religiousness and spirituality in medical rehabilitation and the lives of persons with disabilities. Am J Phys Med Rehabil. 1997;76:255-7.

44a. Schwartz MD, Hughes C, Roth J, et al. Spiritual faith and genetic testing decisions among high-risk breast cancer probands. Cancer Epidemiol Biomarkers Prev. 2000; 9:381-5.

45. Mickley J, Soeken K. Religiousness and hope in Hispanic- and Anglo-American women with breast cancer. Oncol Nurs Forum. 1993;20:1171-7.

46. Juarez G, Ferrell B, Borneman T. Influence of culture on cancer pain management in Hispanic patients. Cancer Practice. 1998;6:262-9.

47. Ali NS. Providing culturally sensitive care to Egyptians with cancer. Cancer Practice. 1996;4:212-5.

48. Trawick M. An Ayurvedic theory of cancer. Med Anthropol. 1991;13:121-36.

49. Luna LJ. Transcultural nursing care of Arab Muslims. J Transcult Nursing. 1989;1:22-6.

50. Alvarado KA, Templer DI, Bresler C, Thomas-Dobson S. The relationship of religious variables to death depression and death anxiety. J Clin Psychol. 1995;51:202-4.

51. Neeleman J, Halpern D, Leon D, Lewis G. Tolerance of suicide, religion and suicide rates: an ecological and individual study in 19 Western countries. Psychol Med. 1997; 27:1165-71.

52. Johnson CJ, McGee MG. How Different Religions View Death and Afterlife. Philadelphia: Charles Press; 1998.

53. Townes EM. Breaking the Fine Rain of Death: African American Health Issues and a Womanist Ethic of Care. New York: Continuum; 1998.

54. Eugene TM. There is a balm in Gilead: black women and the black church as agents of a therapeutic community. Women and Therapy. 1995;16:55-71.

55. Hardy KV, Laszloffy TA. The cultural genogram: key to training culturally competent family therapists. J Marital Fam Ther. 1995;21:227-37.

56. Freeman DL, Abrams JZ, eds. Illness and Health in the Jewish Tradition: Writings from the Bible to Today. Philadelphia: Jewish Publication Society; 1999.

57. Marty M, ed. Health and Medicine in the [Religion] Tradition series. New York: Crossroad. This series discusses several Christian denominations.

58. Rahman F. Health and Medicine in the Islamic Tradition: Change and Identity. New York: Crossroad; 1987.

59. Chopra D. Return of the Rishi: A Doctor's Story of Spiritual Transformation and Ayurvedic Healing. Boston: Houghton Mifflin; 1991.

60. Goleman D, ed. Healing Emotions. Conversations with the Dalai Lama on Mindfulness, Emotions, and Health. Boston: Shambhala; 1997.

61. Arviso Alford L, Cohen Van Pelt E. The Scalpel and the Silver Bear: The First Navajo Woman Surgeon Combines Western Medicine and Traditional Healing. New York: Bantam; 1999.

62. Thao P, Conquergood D (ethnographer), Thao X (translator). I Am a Shaman: A Hmong Life Story With Ethnographic Commentary. Minneapolis: Southeast Asian Refugee Studies Project, Center for Urban and Regional Affairs, University of Minnesota; 1989.

63. Gray J (compiler). Ashe: Traditional Religion and Healing in Sub-Saharan Africa and the Diaspora—A Classified Bibliography. New York: Greenwood Press; 1989.

64. Numbers RL, Amundson DW, eds. Caring and Curing: Health and Medicine in the Western Religious Traditions. New York: Macmillan; 1986.

65. Sullivan L, ed. Healing and Restoring: Health and Medicine in the World's Relgious Traditions. New York: Macmillan; 1989.

66. Martsolf DS. Cultural aspects of spirituality in cancer care. Semin Oncol Nurs. 1997; 13:231-6.

67. Lo B, Quill T, Tulsky J. Discussing palliative care with patients. Ann Intern Med. 1999; 130:744-9.

68. Heliker D. Reevaluation of a nursing diagnosis: spiritual distress. Nursing Forum. 1992; 27:15-20.

69. McKee DD, Chappell JN. Spirituality and medical practice. J Fam Practice. 1992;35: 201,205-8.

70. Leetun MC. Wellness spirituality in the older adult: assessment and intervention protocol. Nurse Pract. 1996; 21:60,65-70.

71. Lukoff D, Lu FG, Turner R. Cultural considerations in the treatment of religious and spiritual problems. Psychiatr Clin North Am. 1995;18:467-85.

72. Turner RP, Lukoff D, Barnhouse RT, Lu FG. Religious or spiritual problem: a culturally sensitive diagnostic category in the DSM-IV. J Nerv Ment Dis. 1995;183:435-44.

73. Kleinman A. Illness meaning and illness behavior. In: McHugh S, Vallis M, eds. Illness Behavior: A Multidisciplinary Model. New York: Plenum Press; 1986:149-60.

74. Sloan RP, Batiella E, VandeCreek L, et al. Should physicians prescribe religious activities? N Engl J Med. 2000;342:1913-6.

75. Sloan RP, VandeCreek L. Letter to the editor. N Engl J Med. 2000;343:1341-2.

9

Advocating for Health Care Systems That Meet the Needs of Diverse Populations

JUDYANN BIGBY, MD

Although the population of the United States has become more diverse, health care leaders have failed to implement adequate policies and procedures to address the needs of all users of the health care system. As a result, not all Americans have equal access to care. The lack of appropriate administrative structures and resources to adequately care for patients from racial, ethnic, linguistic, or other groups that are culturally different from the "average" American can be a source of major frustration and concern for the practicing internist. Though physicians can develop clinical skills to ensure that they are competent to communicate with patients, understand different health beliefs, and acknowledge difference, this effort alone cannot surmount the challenges that are described in this book.

Simply put, the structure of the health care system places significant barriers to access for many minority populations. Thus physicians must concern themselves with what happens *outside* of the individual doctor/patient interaction. Physicians who believe they do not have enough influence to make significant institutional change can reflect on lessons from the Civil Rights movement. Advocacy on the part of individual physicians was instrumental in reversing longstanding legal segregation in hospital facilities and for opening the doors of medical schools to racial and ethnic minorities as well as to women (1,2). There is growing recognition that the health care system itself needs to change in order to address the disparities in access, health status, satisfaction, and quality of care for diverse populations. The care of all patients is likely to improve as a consequence of such efforts.

Standards for Culturally and Linguistically Appropriate Services

The Office of Minority Health (www.omhrc.gov) of the Department of Health and Human Services has developed 14 recommended standards for Culturally and Linguistically Appropriate Services (CLAS). Organized by theme, these standards address culturally competent care, language access services, and organizational supports for cultural competence (Box 9-1). Individual physicians can advocate for developing a strategic plan to address these standards in their individual practices.

Medical practices should strive to systematically incorporate culturally competent principles of care into policies, the administrative structure, and clinical service delivery models. Developing appropriate policies and administrative structures requires planning and monitoring. It is especially appropriate for larger organizations (e.g., practices, medical groups) to have an administrative structure (e.g., work group, task force) that is responsible for these activities. The work group should represent physicians, other professional staff, support staff, and patients if possible. Conducting a cultural competence assessment is an important first step. The results from the assessment should form the basis for articulating short-term and long-term goals and for identifying focused areas for intervention. The work group should also develop specific benchmarks to track progress towards organizational cultural competence (3).

Practically speaking, physicians require specific resources to ensure that they are able to serve diverse populations. If a significant percentage of the population does not speak English and providers are not multilingual, interpreters are necessary to deliver appropriate care. In fact, physicians and institutions that receive federal funds, including Medicare and Medicaid payments, are *obligated* to provide appropriate interpreter services and written materials. Many states also have regulations requiring interpreter services; several states (Washington, Maine, Oregon) have procedures for paying the interpreter. State health departments can provide the physician with complete information. Physicians are also obligated to provide written materials to patients in a language that is appropriate for them. Several organizations post Spanish language materials on their Web sites where materials can be down loaded for free. Check the Office of Minority Health Web site for links or call 800-444-6472.

Tracking Quality of Care and Patient Satisfaction

Most health care organizations collect data for insurers and other parties that monitor quality of care. Tracking quality of care and patient satisfaction are essential to providing culturally competent medical coverage. Health disparities are a potent indication that care is not culturally competent. Individual physicians and practices can use these data to better understand where to concentrate their efforts. To collect data that can be analyzed by race and ethnicity, health care practices need to define the race, ethnic, and language fields, train staff, and require that the proper data be entered for each patient. If criteria of the Health Plan Employer Data and Information Set (HEDIS) are already being used, practices can use these to assess how well they are meeting the standards for each racial and ethnic group and to identify potential disparities. In some instances, national benchmarks for underserved populations have already been described, making it possible to interpret results from an individual practice (4).

Collecting and tracking data alone will not lead to improved quality of care or patient satisfaction. Feedback is required from the patient population. Patients willing to provide an assessment of their care can be invited to participate in focus groups or structured interviews. Strategies for obtaining the general community's perception of the care they receive include asking community members to meet periodically as liaisons between physician and patient groups and meeting periodically with key informants (e.g., religious leaders, health care advocates) from the community.

Physicians can advocate for staff that is reflective of the population served by the clinical site. Staff members who reflect the diversity of the community can help to identify barriers to care and provide insight into how the practice can better accommodate different groups. If there are staff members who are bilingual, avoid using them as interpreters unless they have been specially trained and interpreting is included in their job descriptions. Staff who are pulled away from their jobs to interpret should not have to carry a dual workload or be evaluated on their productivity without taking this into account.

Physicians can advocate for staff time to participate in appropriate training related to the care of diverse populations. Plan follow-up meetings to discuss any important issues that are raised. One-day training sessions are seldom effective in promoting institutional change; in fact, they may lead to increased dissatisfaction because of their limited impact. However,

Box 9-1   Recommended Standards for Culturally and Linguistically Appropriate Health Care Services

PREAMBLE   Culture and language have considerable impact on how patients access and respond to health care services. To ensure equal access to quality health care for diverse populations, health care organizations and providers should:

1. Promote and support the attitudes, behaviors, knowledge, and skills necessary for staff to work respectfully and effectively with patients and each other in a culturally diverse work environment.
2. Have a comprehensive management strategy to address culturally and linguistically appropriate services, including strategic goals, plans, policies, procedures, and designated staff responsible for implementation.
3. Utilize formal mechanisms for community and consumer involvement in the design and execution of service delivery, including planning, policymaking, operations, evaluation, training, and, as appropriate, treatment planning.
4. Develop and implement a strategy to recruit, retain, and promote qualified, diverse, and culturally competent administrative, clinical, and support staff who are trained and qualified to address the needs of the racial and ethnic communities being served.
5. Require and arrange for ongoing education and training for administrative, clinical, and support staff in culturally and linguistically competent service delivery.
6. Provide all patients with limited English proficiency (LEP) access to bilingual staff or interpretation services.
7. Provide written notices, including translated signage at key points of contact, to patients in their primary language informing them of their right to receive interpreter services free of charge.
8. Translate and make available signage and commonly used written patient educational material and other materials for members of the predominant language groups in service areas.
9. Ensure that interpreters and bilingual staff can demonstrate bilingual proficiency and receive training that includes the skills and ethics of interpreting and knowledge in both languages of the terms and concepts relevant to clinical or nonclinical encounters. Because they usually lack these abilities, family members or friends are not considered adequate substitutes.
10. Ensure that each patient's primary spoken language and self-identified race/ethnicity are included in the health care organization's management information system as well as any patient records used by provider staff.

(Cont'd.)

Box 9-1 (continued)

11. Use a variety of methods to collect and analyze accurate demographic, cultural, epidemiologic, and clinical outcome data for racial and ethnic groups in the service area and become informed about the ethnic/cultural needs, resources, and assets of the surrounding community.
12. Undertake ongoing organizational self-assessments of cultural and linguistic competence, and integrate measures of access, satisfaction, quality, and outcomes for culturally and linguistically appropriate services (CLAS) into other organizational internal audits and performance improvement programs.
13. Develop structures and procedures to address cross-cultural ethical and legal conflicts in health care delivery and complaints or grievances by patients and staff about unfair, culturally insensitive, or discriminatory treatment, difficulty in accessing services, and denial of services.
14. Prepare a progress report annually that documents the organization's progress with implementing CLAS standards, including information on programs, staffing, and resources.

From the Office of Minority Health, Public Health Service, United States Department of Health and Human Services.

---

one-day trainings can serve to invigorate people and provide a better understanding of the issues diverse patients face. Physicians can recruit other colleagues to strategize about substantial and long-range interventions to improve cultural competency. Identifying like-minded colleagues is essential for implementing institutional change. Standards and expectations defined by diverse stakeholders are more likely to have a true impact on the process of care that is delivered.

Physicians are in a unique position to advocate for policies and procedures that facilitate care for the populations they are serving. Reviewing policies such as hours of operation, days of operation, registration procedures, strategies for following abnormal tests and procedures, and the way space is arranged can greatly influence access and outcomes. For example, if a practice sees a significant number of Latino patients, it is important to have office space that accommodates an entire family present at a visit to hear about prognosis or updates on a chronic serious condition of the patient. Tracking abnormal tests and compliance with follow-up for Pap smears and mammograms may require different interventions depending on the population served. Some women would not be comfortable with telephone reminders; others may be uncomfortable with registered letters coming to their homes.

Because some racial and ethnic minority populations and some immigrant populations have a high burden of illness, poorer health outcomes, and a higher prevalence of risk factors for chronic disease, "wrap-around" services such as outreach, case management, and health education can help to ensure that patients are engaged in care. Outreach activities facilitate access. Case managers can serve as bridges between health care institutions and as links to appropriate community resources. Providing transportation and extending operating hours may also be required.

True cultural competency implies that physicians are familiar with the population they are serving and can adopt an appropriate population-based clinical practice. Many local health departments can provide basic epidemiologic data about, for example, health status indicators and hospital admission rates. The concept of Community-Oriented Primary Care provides a framework for an approach to individual care that incorporates knowledge of population level data (5).

Cultural competence is a means, not an end. Individual physicians and health care organizations must continuously assess how well they are meeting their goals in achieving cultural competence and adapt their services accordingly to meet the unique needs of different populations. This requires regular reports about each of the activities in place to address culturally competent care and the development of appropriate performance improvement projects. Disparities in health care treatment, satisfaction, and clinical outcomes can be linked to specific improvement projects. Measures that help to improve cultural competence can be incorporated throughout the improvement process.

Getting To Know the Populations Served

Physicians can be visible in the community and learn from their experiences working outside of the health care setting. By developing relationships with community groups such as schools, faith-based organizations, and multiservice providers, physicians can gain new insights into the culture of different groups and the challenges facing them in their communities. Often advocacy groups for different populations hold community-based health fairs or other information sessions. Physicians can volunteer to speak at such events. It is also helpful to invite leaders from the community to speak to staff and create avenues for exchange of information. It is important to integrate what is learned from interacting with the community into the processes of clinical care.

Summary

Health care organizations and practices require several components to deliver culturally competent care. Ideally physicians and other staff should reflect the diversity of the population served. This is not always practicable, but clinical sites should strive to identify opportunities to diversify their clinical and support staffs. If the physicians and staff are not racially or ethnically representative of the community, working together with other practices or groups which are more diverse can facilitate culturally appropriate care.

Clinical practices that value diversity should have diverse representation in its management and policy-making positions. Community representatives should be on governing or advisory boards. Practice policies and procedures should facilitate care for diverse populations. Quality assurance procedures should report outcomes by race/ethnicity, and strategies should be developed to address disparities. Practices should develop benchmarks to track their success in developing culturally competent systems of health care.

REFERENCES

1. Watson WH. Against the Odds: Blacks in the Profession of Medicine in the United States. New Brunswick, NJ: Transaction Publishers; 1999.
2. Bird WM, Clayton LA. An American Health Dilemma: A Medical History of African Americans and the Problem of Race. New York: Routledge; 2002.
3. Checklist for planning, implementing, and evaluating culturally competent service delivery systems in primary health care settings. Community Health Education Manual. Supplement 4, Nov. 2000;35-7.
4. Partridge L, Szlyk CI. National Medicaid HEDIS Database/Benchmark Project: Pilot-Year Experience and Benchmark Results. New York: The Commonwealth Fund; Feb. 2000.
5. Wright RA. Community-oriented primary care: the cornerstone of health reform. JAMA. 1993;269:2544-7.

Index

A

Abortion in Latino culture, 78
Abuse
 alcohol. *See* Alcohol abuse
 in immigrant populations, 217-218
 religion and, 253
Access to health care. *See also* Barrier to
  health care
 by black Americans, 31
 by immigrants, 221, 223, 225
 by Latinos, 66-67, 83-86
Accidental death, 117-118
Acculturation, 217-218
 of Latinos, 67-68
Acquired immunodeficiency syndrome
 in black Americans, 49-50
 in Latino population, 81-82, 88
Acute diarrhea, 204
Advance directive in Arab American
  culture, 189-190
Advocacy for cross-cultural care, 269-275
African American, 29-56. *See also* Black
  American
Age of Latino population, 65-66
Aging, religion and, 255
Airlift, 121
Alaska Native, 96
 cancer in, 117
 health status of, 111-112
 Alcohol abuse
 in American Indian population, 112
 by black Americans, 51-53
 in Latino population, 82
 religion and, 253
Alcoholics Anonymous, 253
Amebic infection, 207-208
American Holistic Medical Association,
  240
American Indian population, 23, 25, 95-
  127
 accidents in, 117-118

American Indian population *(cont'd.)*
 causes of death in, 110-112
 colonial system and, 100-101
 diseases in
  alcoholism in, 112-114
  cancer, 116-117, 124-125
  cardiovascular, 116
  diabetes, 114-116
  pneumonia and influenza, 114
  tuberculosis in, 114
 family structure in, 121-123
 gender roles in, 120-121
 health disparities in, 119
 Indian Health Service and, 106, 110
 Indian-white relations, 96-99
 infant mortality in, 118
 intertribalism and pan-Indianism, 101
 language in, 119-120
 patient-physician relationship in, 123
 suicide in, 118
 violence in, 118
 wellness and unwellness in, 105-106
 world-view of, 101-105
American Muslim. *See* Arab American
  culture
Anesthesia, religious belief and, 254
Antibody, hepatitis, 214
Antigen, hepatitis, 214
Appointment, keeping of
 by Arab American patient, 179
 by Dominican patient, 14-15
Arab American culture, 161-193
 communication in, 175-177
 death and dying in, 187-191
 demographics of, 165-167
 female dress in, 183
 gender roles in, 173
  female segregation and, 181-183
 halaal and *haraam* in, 184-185
 health, illness, and recovery in, 173-175
 hygiene in, 183-184
 immigration patterns of, 164-165

277